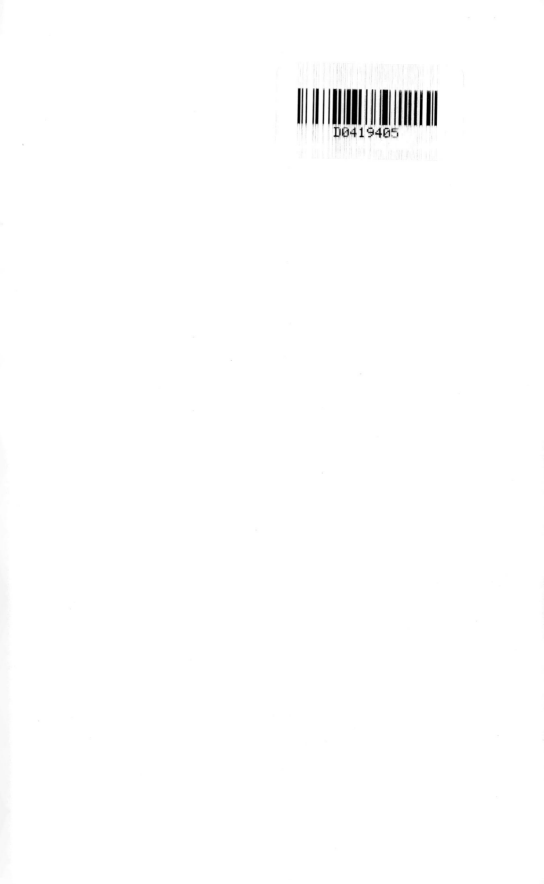

D0419405

Second Edition

Practical Guide to
CLINICAL DATA
MANAGEMENT

Second Edition

Practical Guide to
CLINICAL DATA
MANAGEMENT

Susanne Prokscha

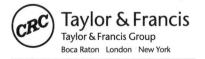

Taylor & Francis
Taylor & Francis Group
Boca Raton   London   New York

CRC is an imprint of the Taylor & Francis Group,
an informa business

CRC Press
Taylor & Francis Group
6000 Broken Sound Parkway NW, Suite 300
Boca Raton, FL 33487-2742

© 2007 by Taylor & Francis Group, LLC
CRC Press is an imprint of Taylor & Francis Group, an Informa business

No claim to original U.S. Government works
Printed in the United States of America on acid-free paper
10 9 8 7 6 5 4 3

International Standard Book Number-10: 0-8493-7615-7 (Hardcover)
International Standard Book Number-13: 978-0-8493-7615-3 (Hardcover)

Library of Congress Cataloging-in-Publication Data

Prokscha, Susanne.
   A practical guide to clinical data management / by Susanne Prokscha. -- 2nd ed.
      p. ; cm.
   Includes bibliographical references and index.
   ISBN 0-8493-7615-7 (Hardcover : alk. paper)
   1. Drugs--Testing--Data processing. 2. Clinical trials--Data processing. 3. Database management. I. Title.
   [DNLM: 1. Database Management Systems--organization & administration. 2. Clinical Trials. 3. Data Collection--methods. 4. Information Management--organization & administration. W 26.55.I4 P964p 2006]

   RM301.27.P76 2006
   615'.19010285--dc22   2006043887

Preface

When new drugs or devices are tested in humans, the data generated by, and related to, these trials are known as clinical data. These data represent a huge investment by the biopharmaceutical or device company and are its greatest assets. It is these data that will eventually make a new product useful, and marketable, in disease therapy. The management of clinical data, from its collection to its extraction for analysis, has become a critical element in the steps to prepare a regulatory submission and to obtain approval to market a treatment. As its importance has grown, clinical data management (CDM) has changed from an essentially clerical task in the late 1970s and early 1980s to the highly computerized specialty it is today.

I wrote the first edition of this book at a time when the role of clinical data managers had developed into a specialty and career. Professional organizations, conferences, and seminars were available but there were few training courses and little information available that dealt with the wide scope of, and variability in, typical data management tasks. The original book was written mainly to provide basic information for new data managers, but it included some more advanced topics for experienced data managers taking on new tasks.

The first edition, written starting in early 1998 and published in 1999, reflected the state of clinical data management and the industry at that time. A new Food and Drug Administration (FDA) regulation, 21 CFR 11, "Electronic Records; Electronic Signatures," had just come into effect at the time of writing and we knew it would have an impact on how clinical data management was carried out, but we did not know the full impact at that point. While data management groups still struggle today in complying with 21 CFR 11, the basic requirements and expectations are now fairly clear. This new edition incorporates the changes that data management groups have made under 21 CFR 11 and also the other changes that I have seen in data management industry practices. The FDA, industry auditors, and directors of data management groups all have higher expectations now for how data management tasks are carried out. This book is meant to help data managers understand those expectations.

Another big change that has taken place since the first edition has been the move to *much* greater use of electronic data capture (EDC) in place of standard paper case report forms. At the time of this writing, most companies are at a minimum experimenting with EDC and some will perform only EDC trials. In revising each chapter, I looked for opportunities to point out differences (and similarities) in data management between EDC-based studies and paper-based studies. At this time, all data managers have to understand processing for both types of studies.

To address the new expectations and reflect the kind of work that data managers typically see today, the book has been reorganized. Part I, "Elements of the Process," covers the basic data management tasks that all data managers must understand and all data management groups must deal with. Part II, "Necessary Infrastructure," is new. It addresses the expectations of the FDA and auditors for how data management groups carry out their work in compliance with regulations. Part III, "CDM Systems," focuses on the computer systems, including EDC, that all data management groups use and the special procedures that must be in place to support those systems.

Even though industry and FDA expectations for quality in data management are higher, that still does not mean that there is only one way to do things. Often, there are several perfectly acceptable ways to perform a task, any of which would ensure the integrity of the data and the ability to analyze it. To acknowledge this diversity, every chapter presents a range of successful and, above all, practical options for each element of the process or task. This by no means implies that the approaches presented here are the only possible ones! One thing I have learned is that there are always new ways to tackle a task, and one has to understand the complete environment (human and technical) to define an approach that will work best for a given situation. The key to finding a successful, practical approach to data management tasks in any environment is to be aware of the range of possibilities and the implications of each. That is the aim of this book: to provide data managers with enough background information and a number of options for a task so they can find or develop an approach that gets the work done with efficiency and quality.

Susanne Prokscha

The Author

Susanne Prokscha is an independent consultant in clinical data management specializing in supporting the many small and emerging companies on the West Coast. She earned a degree in physics from the Massachusetts Institute of Technology in 1981 and went on to do graduate work at Brandeis University. On leaving graduate school, she worked as a staff physicist for a medical device manufacturer and became interested in clinical data and clinical trials. She has held a variety of senior consulting positions at software vendors and service providers both in the United States and in Europe since the mid-1980s. She has been an independent consultant since January 2001.

Ms. Prokscha's work with a large variety of companies led her to write the first edition on the process of data management: *Practical Guide to Clinical Data Management* (Interpharm Press, 1999). She is often called upon to give seminars and training sessions for data management professionals through the Drug Information Association, Society for Clinical Data Managers, and other organizations. She is also an instructor for the extension programs of the University of California Berkeley and the University of California Santa Cruz.

Contents

part one

Elements of the process

In the first part of this book, we cover the elements or steps of the data management process that are nearly universal. Any data management group, large or small, long established, or just emerging, will have to perform these tasks or be closely involved with them. Even companies that do not perform data management in house, but rather send all their data management work to contract research organizations, will need to beware of these elements and oversee them as they are carried out.

chapter one

The data management plan

From the time that data management groups were first formed, they set up studies, collected or entered data, cleaned those data, and processed them until the study could be considered ready for analysis. For the most part, they all did a good job of this and produced datasets with accurate data that reflected values provided by the investigator sites. Over time, as the idea of "if you didn't document it, it wasn't done" became the rule, groups made an effort to produce documents at key points along the way to record what was done and to provide evidence of good practice. These documents were (and still are) filed together in what is frequently referred to simply as the "study file." To ensure that study files across groups were consistent, these companies eventually wrote standard operating procedures (SOPs) that outlined what the contents of each study file should be.

However, even with good study files, some data management groups found they could not always quickly find an answer when an auditor asked a specific question about the conduct of a past study. So, several years ago, some companies began to address this problem by creating a document whose purpose was to record all the most important information on how data management was carried out for a study. They quickly found that creating this kind of document at the start of a study provides added value — beyond its function as a reference — by forcing study planning. The documents are also more accurate when written at the start of a study rather than as a summary or report at the end of the study. This kind of document is called a "data management plan" (DMP). (Another common name for this document is "data handling plan.") In recent years, this type of document has become an industry standard practice. If an auditor looks into a company's data management activities, that auditor will generally begin by asking for the DMP for a given study.

A DMP that is written at the beginning of a study provides a focus for identifying the work to be performed, who will perform that work, and what is to be produced as documentation of the work. Plans can vary in length depending on the size of the data management group and how standard study activities are. A DMP may be a bulleted list of items covering a few pages, a thick document with an index, or something in between. In this chapter, we will discuss what goes into these plans and how to use them efficiently.

What goes into a plan?

A DMP should touch on all the elements of the data management process for the study in question. The elements are those that form the structure of Part I of this book and are summarized in Figure 1.1. For each element or group of elements in the data management process, a DMP specifies:

- What is the work to be performed?
- Who is responsible for the work?
- Which SOPs or guidelines will apply?
- What documentation or output will be collected or produced?

By including the final point in each section, that of documentation or output, the DMP also becomes an approximate table of contents for the study file and can be used as a source document for internal quality assurance audits.

There is a lot of consistency in the content of DMPs from company to company. DMPs across companies touch on roughly the same topics, even if the exact names of the headers or the ways the topics are grouped into sections vary. However, experienced data managers can still differ quite a lot in their opinions as to how much detail to include in a particular section of a DMP. At some companies, the DMP is very detailed and includes text copied from other documents so that the plan is a complete record of the study. More commonly, the DMP documents key information not included elsewhere and refers to appendices or other independent documents for details. Both of these approaches are valid and meet the need of consolidating data management process information.

Topics to Cover in a Data Management Plan

---

1. CRF design
2. Study setup
3. Tracking CRF data (CRF workflow)
4. Entering data
5. Cleaning data
6. Managing lab data
7. SAE handling
8. Coding reported terms
9. Creating reports and transferring data
10. Closing studies

Figure 1.1 Elements of the data management process that should be addressed in a data management plan.

An example of one DMP template, or outline, can be found in Appendix A. This outline can be used for nearly all kinds of studies at all kinds of companies.

Revising the DMP

It is very likely that during the course of an average study, some critical data management process or a key computer application will change. Even in a short-term study, some detail of a data handling procedure or a number of cleaning checks will change as the group acquires experience with the data specific to that trial. Even though the DMP is a *plan*, that is, it is the way you expect to conduct the study, it must be revised whenever there is a significant change because it will then show how you expect to conduct the study from that point forward. The DMP must be kept current, and that is harder to manage than one might expect.

Companies constantly wrestle with finding the best or most practical way to record updates to the data management process in a DMP. When reviewing or creating a DMP-revision process, a company should consider these points:

- How "big" a change must it be to appear as a revision in the DMP? Is normal change control sufficient or does it warrant attention in the plan?
- If a document referred to in the DMP is updated, does its version number have to be updated in the DMP?
- If an appendix is updated, does the DMP, as a whole, require a revision with a new version number?
- Who needs to sign off on revisions?

In whatever way it is accomplished, after study lock, the DMP should reflect all important changes to the data management process and computer systems that took place during the study.

Using plans with CROs

When a sponsor uses a contract research organization (CRO) to conduct all or part of the data management activities for a study, either the sponsor's or the CRO's DMP can be used. Many companies, especially smaller companies, will use the CRO's DMP. In fact, many CROs have more comprehensive plans than those found at sponsors because they hold themselves to a higher level of documentation for their process. An experienced data manager from the sponsor company should expect to review in detail, and sign off on, the CRO's DMP. The CRO should explain what the process will be for revising the DMP during the course of the study. It is the sponsor's responsibility to allocate resources to get the initial DMP and all revisions reviewed and signed in a reasonable period of time.

Quality assurance and DMPs

Quality assurance (QA) is the prevention, detection, and correction of errors or problems. In biopharmaceutical firms, QA is closely tied to regulatory compliance because good practice must be closely tied to following regulations. Regulatory compliance and quality assurance are critical even in emerging companies too small to have a separate QA group. A key requirement of most quality methods is the creation of a plan; a key requirement of Good Clinical Practice (GCP) is the documentation of what has happened during a study. The DMP helps fulfill both of these requirements by creating the plan and detailing what documents will record the conduct of the study. The DMP and the output documents it requires can be used as the starting point when conducting internal QA audits of the data management process. As noted above, it is also used by external auditors.

SOPs for DMPs and study files

Every data management group should have a process for documenting how a study was conducted. The process must be described formally in either an SOP or a department guideline. For most companies, this means that they will require a DMP for each study. Some companies will address this need by creating a detailed SOP governing the contents of the study file.

For companies that require a DMP, the requirement should cover in-house studies as well as those conducted by a CRO. The procedure should be clear at which point the plan must be in place. For the DMP to be a *plan* — rather than a *report* at the end of the study — a draft or an initial version typically needs to be in place before any substantial data management work is performed for the study. A section on the requirements for revision control of the document should clearly state under what circumstances the DMP must be revised and how the revision is to be documented. Along with the procedure for creating and maintaining a DMP, there should be a blank template document or an outline for the plan to assure consistency. Each section in the template should have instructions on what kind of information and what level of detail is expected. An example of a completed DMP is also a good way to show the level of detail expected by a given company.

DMPs specify what output documents are to be created during the course of the study. These must be filed somewhere. The details of the study file may be described in a separate SOP or covered in the DMP SOP. In either case, the two must be kept in synchronization. If the SOP for the DMP states that the final database design will be filed in the study file, there must be a folder or tab in the study file for that document. Many companies make the mistake of letting the study file and DMP requirements drift apart so that an auditor will see that a particular folder is required by the SOP, but the contents will be blank because the DMP no longer requires that output. Always be very careful in using the word "require" in an SOP. If the SOP states that the study file *must* have a particular folder or tab, it must actually be there — with something in it — during an audit. Require only those folders you actually require; use more vague text such as "may include" for others.

Companies that use only study files, not a DMP document, will have only a study file SOP but will still collect the same information. All information required to document the conduct of the study should be listed in the study file SOP. The same issues noted above apply here as well: be careful what you require, and if you require it, make sure it is actually in the study file when it is supposed to be filed.

Finally, for both approaches, consider how to file documents for CRO studies. Some documents normally produced during a study conducted by the sponsor may be produced by the CRO as well but are then kept internally by the CRO rather than transferred to the sponsor. One example is a CRF annotated for the database design. If the sponsor will receive transfer datasets at the end of study (rather than a database transfer of some sort), the sponsor has no need of this design document for the database. For each study and sponsor/CRO combination there will be issues like this. One option is to have a different list of study-file requirements for CRO studies; having the same set of folders or tabs and slipping a "not applicable" note into many of them is another option.

Using data management plans

To overcome the natural, strong reluctance to spend time planning or documenting anything when there is "real" work to be done, the value of the effort must be recognized. To get more than minimal compliance from staff, that value has to be more than "because so-and-so tells us we have to" or "the FDA requires it." A DMP actually does have benefits that can be recognized by every data manager. These benefits include:

- The work to be done and responsibilities are clearly stated at the start of the study so that everyone knows what is expected.
- The expected documents are listed at the start of the study so they can be produced during the course of, rather than after, the conduct of the study.
- The document helps everyone fulfill regulatory requirements.
- Data management tasks become more visible to other groups when the DMP is made available to the project team.
- The DMP provides continuity of process and a history of a project. This is particularly useful for long-term studies and growing data management groups.

Forcing the planning work to take place at the beginning of the study may be hard, but it will save time at the close of the study when the time pressure likely will be even stronger. To avoid overwhelming staff with documentation requirements, managers of data management groups should encourage the use of templates and the use of previous plans. The first few plans will require some work; after that the burden should be considerably reduced as each new plan builds on the experience of the previous ones. The key is to keep DMP requirements both focused and practical.

chapter two

CRF design considerations

Paper case report forms (CRFs) or electronic forms (eCRFs) for use in electronic data capture systems are developed along with, or shortly after, the development of the clinical protocol to reflect the needs of the protocol in collecting the appropriate data for analysis. At some companies, the first draft of the CRF is created by a clinical research associate; at others, data managers prepare the initial version. Even if data managers are not responsible for the creation of the CRF, they should be closely involved in its review and approval as part of a cross-functional team.

A cross-functional team is the only way to design a CRF that will collect the necessary data in a way that is clear and easy for the investigator, efficient for data management processing, and appropriate for analysis. The team must balance company standards with the needs of the individual study and take into account preferences of the team members and investigators. In weighing needs and preferences, the final deciding question must be: "Can the data from the CRF be analyzed to make decisions about safety and efficacy?"

Data managers can find several useful sources of guidelines for the *layout* of fields on the CRF, but information on the implications of layout choices on data management is less widely available and forms the focus of this chapter. For the most part, the issues and concepts that follow apply to both paper CRFs and entry screens that are part of electronic data capture applications. The first topic in this chapter, "Data Cleaning Issues," will cover CRF designs that impact data cleaning and site queries (see also Chapter 7, "Cleaning Data"). The second topic, "Data Processing Issues," will address CRF designs that impact how data is entered and stored (see also Chapter 3, "Database Design Considerations"). Later in the chapter we will also look at handling revisions to CRFs and general quality considerations.

9

Data cleaning issues

Discrepancies in data is time-consuming to identify, track, and resolve — especially when they involve a query to a site. Therefore, working on a CRF design that reduces the need for checks on fields that are administrative only (that is, they do not actually add to the quality of the data) has a lot of value to data management. Asking the investigator to provide duplicate or repeat information in different locations is one such source of low-value queries. Other low-value queries will be generated if the CRF designer does not make adequate provision for blank or unavailable responses or permits ambiguous responses.

Duplicate data

CRFs frequently include questions that are intentionally used as cross-checks to other fields. This can be a very good policy when the data is actually different. For example, cleaning programs can check for logical consistency by comparing the sex of the patient to the patient's pregnancy status. Or, the weight of a patient can be checked against a weight-dependent dosage to assure proper compliance with the protocol. The fields are different, but related.

Problems do arise, however, when cleaning programs cross-check values that are actually duplicates of the same data. For example, a CRF should not ask for both the patient's age and birth date. Data management or analysis software can easily calculate the patient's age from the birth date, or just the age can be used. Discrepancies and confusion are bound to be generated when the investigator asks for both values and they do not agree. Similarly, CRFs should avoid questions that ask an investigator to repeat values such as "Time of treatment start" in multiple fields, even on the same page, or request that values from one page be copied to another without good justification. The values will *have* to be checked against each other and mismatches will, without a doubt, occur.

A form of indirect duplication of values in the CRF is asking the investigator to calculate values. If the protocol asks the investigator to measure blood pressure three times and then to calculate the mean, the value of the mean may be inappropriately duplicating the information in the three measurements. As with the example of age and birth date, a computer can easily calculate the mean and would avoid discrepancies caused by miscalculation on the investigator's part. Sometimes a protocol does require the investigator to perform calculations as part of determining the correct course of treatment. In this case, the trial sponsor should consider providing space and methods for the calculation on a worksheet or in an instruction area that is not entered as part of the CRF data. A monitor would double-check the calculation as part of the normal source document verification.

It is worth noting, having warned against it, at least one example of a case when duplication does provide value in data cleaning. Header information, such as patient identifiers and initials, are such an example of useful duplication.

CRFs usually repeat header sections on each page. In studies where pages can come in singly or become separated from the booklet, a cross-check of patient ID with initials for the data on every page against enrollment information has proven invaluable in identifying mislabeled pages.

Missing and ambiguous responses

Missing and ambiguous responses can occur at the level of the individual field, at the level of a module (or grouping of questions) on the CRF, or at the entire page level. When considering CRF layout, the design team should consider appropriate actions at each level.

Field level

Questions on a CRF should generally not allow "Blank" to be an expected response. For example, if a number of possible symptoms are listed on the page and the instructions are to "Check the box if yes," then a "No" response would leave a box blank. If none of the boxes in that section are checked, there is no way of knowing if the response was "No" for each symptom or if they were inadvertently overlooked by the site. Data management might annoy the investigator sites by double-checking via a query. It is always better to include the full range of replies in these cases, including a "Not applicable," if appropriate.

For CRF fields that are not associated with check boxes, data management, working together with clinical and biostatistics team members, should decide whether or not to instruct the sites to write something in a field if there is no data or reply available. Common indicators that the response for a field is not available include: NA (not applicable), ND (not done), or UNK (unknown). The team must decide if only one or a selection of these texts is to be deemed an acceptable response. In some data management groups, the text is actually entered into the database for that field (or into a related text field; see Chapter 3 for more on this), in which case no discrepancy is raised. In other groups, data entry staff leave the fields blank when the site indicates "NA." A discrepancy will be raised because there is no value in the field, but the data manager reviewing the discrepancy will see that the site indicated the value as NA and will close the discrepancy without issuing a query to the site.

Module level

While a single missing value here and there is to be expected, it is also worthwhile to make accommodations for an entire set of questions to have no responses. When questions on a page are logically connected, they are usually grouped into a set and often visually linked via a box around the group. This is frequently known as a CRF "module." If it is at all possible that the site will have no responses for the entire module (and this usually means it could happen to any module), it is worthwhile having a not-done box at the start of the module. If the not-done box is checked, no discrepancies will be raised when the values are blank.

Page level

The module not-done box can be taken up a level because ambiguity of missing values can also occur at the page level. For example, some adverse event (AE) forms have a header section followed directly by the fields used to report AE data. If that page comes in to data management with all header information filled in but the rest blank, there is no way of knowing if there were no AEs or if the page was inadvertently left blank. Other types of important data, such as concomitant medications, have the same characteristics. It would be unusual for a site to fill in NA for a page like this.

These kinds of pages or modules should have an "indicator field" after the header that asks "Were there any adverse events?" (or medications, or whatever). To be consistent with the suggestion above, the indicator variable should have a full set of yes/no boxes to check as the response.

Data processing issues

Certain kinds of CRF page designs may be necessary and appropriate but still have a significant impact on the way the study is processed. When reviewing CRFs, data managers should keep an eye out for these kinds of page designs and plan for their impact — not just on one particular data value or set of values but also on the flow of the data through the process. Examples of designs that impact processing include:

- Comments or longer free texts
- Diagrams or analog scales
- "Log" type forms for (AEs), etc.
- Patient questionnaires
- Early termination pages

Comments

As we will see in Chapter 3, "Database Design Considerations," long text fields have a considerable impact on database design. The text in long comment fields is rarely analyzed and is most frequently used during manual review by monitors or others in the clinical team to cross-check against other problems reported or found in the data. The length of the text can pose a serious problem for the database designer because some databases have limits on the length of ordinary text fields. However, if the comment appears in a CRF it must be stored either in the database along with other CRF values or on an image linked to the database information.

Long and also short text comments impact not only design choices but also normal processing. If the data is being transcribed into a database through double entry, comment fields can really slow down the effort. Even small variations in the way a comment text is entered (e.g., line breaks, spaces) can cause the two entries not to match. This can be a significant enough problem that some companies opt for a visual verification of comment texts rather than a character for character comparison. In systems using optical character recognition (OCR) as a first entry pass (see Chapter 5), the OCR engine usually is not used on text at all — much less on longer comments. These are entered manually in a second-review pass after OCR and, as in the case of double entry, this significantly adds to the processing effort.

Longer texts also increase the chance of encountering illegible handwriting and the annoying question of misspellings. Many data management groups resort to a manual listing review of all comment or longer text fields to identify unusual entries — and whether they came from the site or the entry staff. With all the additional resources and processing needed to make text or comment fields contain quality data with some value, CRF designers should keep such fields to a minimum!

Diagrams and analog scales

Some studies collect information in areas such as disease history and efficacy using diagrams or analog scales. Data from either of these can be very tedious to transcribe into a database. In the case of diagrams, it may not be possible to summarize the information in a form that can be stored in a typical database.

Diagrams might be preprinted or hand-drawn representations. A human figure on which the investigator marks affected areas is an example of a preprinted diagram. A hand-drawn example would be a box in which the investigator sketches a representation of a rash or tumor. Both methods allow the investigator to provide very specific details as to the location or condition in question. Collecting the information from a preprinted diagram for storage in a database may involve categorizing the figure into sections and having a clinical research associate CRA or data management enter section identifiers. Collecting information from hand-drawn diagrams may involve identifying certain parameters of interest and taking measurements to provide the data for those parameters. Most typically, companies recognize that the data only can be analyzed by a human as a complete image and not to try to quantify the data. Because of the problems associated with obtaining information from them, diagrams are not commonly found on CRF pages.

Analog scales, however, are very common. An analog scale is a line with two extremes described at each end. The patient makes a mark on the line to indicate the appropriate level between the extremes allowing patients to indicate exactly how they feel. The continuous scale avoids forcing a patient to fit their responses into a predetermined set of categories such as "mild, moderate, or severe." Analog scales are often used in quality-of-life-type questions, such as an indication of a patient's level of pain or of the level of satisfaction with a given treatment.

Capturing the data from analog scales usually entails measuring the point at which the patient's mark crosses the line. Sometimes the line is of a fixed length, and the distance from the low extreme (e.g., zero) to the patient's mark provides the data value. To work across patients, the length has to be exactly the same for each patient. In cases where the length of the scale may vary (as it may when certain kinds of printing are used), two measurements are made: that of the length of the entire line and that of the position of the mark. The person making the measurement must be very careful and the rulers must all be exactly the same. Frequently, the site or the monitor will be asked to make the measurement and record the number on the CRF. In some cases, however, data entry will make the measurement and enter it. In this case, it is critical the actual measurement be verified, not just the entry of the result into the database.

Electronic CRFs and other electronic patient-recorded outcome (PRO) tools can handle both preprinted diagrams and analog scales extremely well. The investigator makes a mark on a diagram or a patient marks a point on a scale and the computer stores a resulting data value. No rulers or grids are needed. All data management departments should consider using these tools for diagrams or scales in large trials — even if the rest of the data is collected on a paper CRF. Note, however, in the case of analog scales, many experts insist that the scale must appear exactly the same to the patient each time it is presented and it must appear the same to all patients. The application cannot scale the analog scale to the display screen size of various computers!

Log forms

Most CRF pages collect information associated with one particular visit or treatment round. For some applications, summary CRF pages that collect information across visits make sense. Many companies call these kinds of forms "log forms." The investigator enters information on that page as the study progresses, completing the page with the final data as the patient completes the study or as the page is filled up. These log forms are used because they have advantages for certain types of data — but they have an impact on how the data is processed. Data management must be aware of the advantages and implications.

AE and concomitant medications are good examples of the kind of data that can be collected sensibly either with a visit-treatment-based form or with a log form. In a visit-treatment-based version of a concomitant medication form, the data collected on a page is the list of concomitant medications for that visit/treatment or since the last collection only. There are usually some medications that are continuing from the last time, some that have started and stopped, and some that have newly started and are continuing. When analysis of this kind of data is made to determine interactions with other medications or the relationship with reported AEs, statisticians try to collapse all the reports into a single list of start and stop times. This turns out to be difficult. Patients and investigators have a hard time keeping the continuing medications straight from visit/treatment to visit/treatment. Some are forgotten; others described differently so that it is not clear whether or not they match up with a previously noted medication. On a log form version, the concomitant medications are listed independent of visit, with just their start and end times or an indication that they are continuing past the end of the study. This does away with the problems of collapsing the data into a single, coherent list. Adverse event log forms have similar advantages in collapsing events.

The difficulty with log forms centers on when they come in to data management. Most are designed to come in at the end of treatment or at the end of the study — in which case a significant amount of work is needed to enter the information, code it, and check for and resolve discrepancies. Log forms will also show up as "expected" or "missing" on CRF completion reports until at least one page comes in. Most importantly, all this critical data is on paper until it comes in and not in the database.

At some companies, early versions of the log forms are sent in as a fax or copy as the study proceeds. This allows for data entry and discrepancy checking of the available data. Unfortunately, data entry staff must be trained to enter any new data and also to check the previously entered data to see if anything has changed each time the page arrives. One approach to dealing with these entry issues is to perform first entry on the data when it first comes in and then to do a final, second entry pass of the entire set when the final version arrives. While this method assures that the data and the final version agree, not all data entry applications support this kind of partial entry very well.

For recording medication or events that may be ongoing through the course of the study, both log forms and visit-treatment-based forms have advantages and disadvantages. The cross-functional design team is the right place to discuss the impact of both types of forms and decide on an appropriate approach for a given company or study.

Questionnaires

Quality-of-life questionnaires introduce interesting considerations to the data management process. Questionnaires are to be filled out by the patient during a visit to the site. Even in studies conducted solely in the United States, these questionnaires will be offered in languages other than English. Typically the questionnaire CRF pages will be sent out to a certified translator. The least impact on the data management process can be achieved if the translator is instructed to keep the same questions on the same page. That is, if questions 1 through 10 appear on the first page in the English version, questions 1 through 10 should appear on the first page in the Spanish version. This will allow the CRF pages to have the same page number and for the entry screens to remain the same. The entry staff will simply enter the responses indicated by the patient regardless of the language used to ask the question. When a site requests a special language version of the questionnaires, they simply swap out the English pages for the customized pages. Tracking and missing page reports need not be changed.

When the translated questions do not map to the same pages, the impact to database design, entry screens, cleaning programs, and tracking will be huge. To facilitate the translations, CRF designers should keep the English language versions fairly sparse as other many languages require a longer text length to convey the same meaning. Note that data management groups should consult with clinical and biostatistics team members to determine whether there is value in storing the language of the questionnaire that is the source of the data for any given patient.

Early termination visits

Except perhaps for Phase I studies, it is likely that some patients will leave a study before they complete the course of visits or treatment. Leaving a study early is commonly called "early termination." Clinical protocols typically include instructions to the sites on what to do if a patient terminates early. The protocol will provide the instructions in the form of which tests should be performed, what samples should be taken, and what additional information is to be gathered. The CRF designers are left to translate that into CRF pages.

Because the protocol instructions are often of the form "in the case of early termination, the patient should fulfill the requirements associated with the Day 50 visit, as well as the study drug and study termination pages...." the CRF designer may choose to designate the pages associated with Day 50 (in this example) as "Day 50 or Early Termination." Unfortunately, while this does meet the requirements of the study, it has a negative impact on the data. In this case, it may not be possible to determine whether the data came from Day 50 or from an Early Termination visit once it is in the database! The question is further confounded if the patient did, in fact, complete the visit prior to Day 50 and then terminated early. If the patient goes past Day 50 and then terminates, there will be two sets of data for Day 50. While all this can be clarified at the end of the study by manual inspection, it will impact discrepancies, CRF tracking, and lab data received from central labs during the course of the study.

A separate set of Early Termination pages may add to the amount of paper sent to the site or the number of eCRF screens that have to be developed but it will result in much clearer data and easier processing during the course of the study. The Early Termination pages may be a full set of pages including the specific study termination forms, or they may be only those pages needed to collect data in addition to the normal study termination forms. The choice between those two approaches will be influenced by specific data management and CRF tracking systems being used for a given study.

Revisions to the CRF

During the course of the study, a clinical protocol may change in such a way as to impact the CRF pages. Two common changes are the addition of lab tests and changes to the inclusion or exclusion criteria. Whenever a revision to a page is required, the data management group, together with the clinical team members, must evaluate the appropriate course of action and thoroughly understand the implications of the change. It may be worth creating a "change document" for each CRF change that evaluates:

- What to do about pages already containing data — must they be transcribed?
- Will both old and new pages will come in, or will blank pages be swapped out at the site?
- What is the impact on the database — must items be added or removed, or do only entry screens require changes?
- How are data cleaning rules affected — do we need to add, delete, or modify cleaning rules?
- How about existing data — are any manual queries required to confirm previously received data based in light of new requirements?

It is fairly common for a question to arise after a CRF change regarding which version of a CRF page was used by a site for a given patient. Consider storing the page version information in one of the systems being used in data management. This may be the clinical database, an associated imaging system, or the CRF tracking system, as appropriate but note that statistical programmers like having the version number with the data in the database for studies where the CRF changes impact how the data will be reported.

Quality assurance for CRFs

The best form of quality assurance for CRF design may be having experienced members of the CRF team carefully review each page and also sign off on the design. As a team, or as individuals, they should be checking:

- That all tests and data required by the protocol are found at the appropriate visit.
- That the data to be used in analysis is actually being collected.
- That standard or historical CRF modules have been used, if they are available.
- That checklists or codes for categorical fields are consistent within this study and across related studies.
- That instructions printed on the CRF are clear and unambiguous.

Many companies also find it useful to have a CRF reviewed by a medical writer or editor who will look for consistent formatting as well as misspellings.

SOPs on CRF design

An SOP on CRF design will likely be a cross-functional one approved by all groups involved. The content of the SOP can be fairly light — perhaps only outlining the expected flow from who is responsible for initiating and/or leading the process through all the people who will sign off on a final version. As always, there must be a procedure in place for amending a CRF page and approving that amendment.

Reuse and refine CRF modules

Companies, not just data management groups, benefit from the use of standard modules for CRF design. When a standard module is used, the completion instructions are the same, the database design is the same, the edit checks are the same, and the associated listing and analysis programs are the same. It is also easier to compare or combine data across studies that use standard forms. That being said, a very common problem that companies face is not changing a module when it is not working! If data management has found problems processing data from a certain CRF module, it is the group's responsibility to take that into consideration and refine the module for the next study.

chapter three

Database design considerations

Data from a clinical trial will be collected and stored in some kind of computer system. The initial data capture method may be paper, a computer entry screen at the investigator's site, a laboratory instrument, central lab system, or perhaps a hand-held computer used to collect diary information from the patient. Regardless of the way the data is captured initially, it must eventually be collected and stored in a computer system or systems that will allow complex data cleaning, reviewing, and reporting. The storage and maintenance of data is achieved by getting it into one or more databases. (A database is simply a structured set of data. This may be an Excel spreadsheet, a Microsoft Access application, an indexed proprietary data format, a collection of SAS tables, or a set of tables built in one of the traditional relational applications such as Oracle®.)

For any software that a company uses to store and manage clinical data, the data manager will design structures, a database, for each clinical trial after the protocol has been defined and the capture methods (such as case report form [CRF] booklets or electronic data capture [EDC] entry screens) have been drafted. A discussion of the design of the main capture methods can be found in Chapter 2. This chapter focuses on the design considerations that go into translating a CRF or protocol into a database for storage, cleaning, and later analysis of the data. The chapter that follows this one, Chapter 4, discusses the steps involved in putting design decisions into action: setup, building, and release of a study.

Making design decisions

No matter what the underlying database or software application, the main design goal for all databases containing information from clinical trials is to store the data accurately. Beyond accuracy, a good database design balances various needs, preferences, and limitations such as:

19

- Clarity, ease, and speed of data entry
- Efficient creation of analysis data sets for biostatisticians
- Formats of data transfer files
- Database design theory
- Database application software requirements

to come up with a practical database. Balance is really the key word, and preference is typically given to designs that make frequent tasks or those requiring highly trained (expensive) staff the easiest to work with.

Often there are several different ways of approaching a database structure design for a given study, *all of which are perfectly valid and technically possible.* One biopharmaceutical firm may choose structures that speed entry; another may choose structures that require less transformation to create analysis data sets. One company may choose to load data from electronic files as-is to avoid complex remapping; another may reformat to be consistent with best practices for database design. In addition, when balancing company needs and preferences, all designs have to allow for the constraints imposed by the software applications that actually manage the clinical database.

As noted above, the design of a database always follows creation of the protocol document. The protocol defines what data is to be collected and on what visit schedule. This could provide enough information to create a database design; however, most companies define the data capture instruments before the database. Data capture instruments are the means of collecting the data from the site. CRF pages or electronic data entry screens are the most common means of data collection, but other sources may include lab data files, integrated voice response (IVR) systems, and so forth. Because they collect data from the sites, the data capture instruments should be carefully designed to be clear and easy to use. In most (but not all) systems, the definition of a data collection device influences, but *does not* completely determine, the design of the database.

The fact that the data collection instrument does not completely define the database storage structures is critical. Data from a given CRF page or electronic file can often be stored in a variety of ways in a database. All data managers, whether or not they are responsible for creating a database design from scratch, should understand the kinds of fields and organization of fields that affect storage, analysis, and processing of the trial data, and they should be aware of some of the options to weigh in making a design decision for those fields.

High-impact fields

Some kinds of data or fields have a higher impact on data management than others. These kinds of fields include:

- Hidden text fields, where text appears along with numeric values
- Dates of all kinds

- Text fields and annotations
- Header information
- Single check boxes
- Calculated or derived values
- Special integers

Hidden text fields

Text in numeric fields occurs in all kinds of studies and in all kinds of clinical data and creates a tension between the need to record exactly what is on the CRF and the need to collect data that actually can be analyzed in a sensible way. Examples of this type of data include: the word "trace" found among lab measurements, a value of "<5" found in an efficacy measure, or a range of "10–15" found in a count of lesions. With assistance from clinical staff, data managers must identify which fields may contain data like this and decide on a storage option. Options for handling this type of data include:

- Design the database field to be a text field so that both numeric and text values can be entered. At the time of analysis, the values that can be converted to numeric will be. Be aware that this may limit the kinds of field level checking that are possible.
- Use a numeric field to store the data and issue a discrepancy if there is text in the field. This makes the most sense when the data represents a critical measurement expected to be numeric.
- Create two fields: one text and one numeric. All data from the CRF is entered in the text field. The values in the second, numeric, field would be automatically derived from the first when the first contains numeric values. Data cleaning is performed only on the numeric value.
- Use a numeric field to store the numeric values and create an associated text or comment field to hold text values when they appear. The investigator (if using remote entry) or the data entry staff must know to use the second field.
- Set data entry guidelines so that a numeric value is chosen. "Trace" may be entered as "0," "<5" as "4," and "10–15" as "13" (midpoint of range).

Different fields may warrant different approaches. It is not necessary to pick an option and apply it to all of these kinds of fields in a study! Consult with both clinical experts and statisticians to make appropriate choices.

Dates

Dates seem to be a clearly defined data type that should not cause problems for data management. However, problems arise constantly with incomplete dates and varying date formats. An example of an incomplete date is when the value is given as "6/-/95" for June 1995 instead of a specific date such as

June 12, 2001. European dates of the form "dd.mm.yyyy" are the classic example of different ways of expressing a date, but even in the United States some sites will use "mm/dd/yyyy" and others will use "dd-mon-yyyy." The majority of database applications do not have good handling of partial dates, nor can they handle a variety of formats in the same study. Therefore, the database design must take the possibility of incomplete dates and also different formats into account.

Dates on a CRF typically fall into three categories:

1. Known dates related to the study (visit date, lab sample date)
2. Historical dates (previous surgery, prior treatment)
3. Dates closely related to the study but provided by the patient (concomitant medication, adverse events [AEs])

The first kind of date is needed for proper analysis of the study, and adherence to the protocol, and so in theory, should always be complete. The second kind of date is often not exactly known to the patient and so partial dates are common. The last type is particularly difficult because the dates are actually useful but not always known exactly, especially if there is a significant time span between visits.

A normal database data type of date usually works just fine for known dates related to the study. If the date is incomplete, nothing is stored in the database, a discrepancy can be issued, and it is likely a full resolution can be found. Dates in the second category are frequently not analyzed but are collected and stored for reference and medical review. A good option for these kinds of dates is a simple text field that would allow dates of any kind.

The third category of dates presents data management with many problems. These dates may be used for analysis, and so they should be complete, but the patient may not know the exact full date. A few companies have had data entry staff fill in the missing date parts according to entry guidelines. Unfortunately, this has resulted in inconsistencies and misunderstanding. More typically, companies address this problem by creating three separate fields for the month, day, and year, and have a fourth, derived, field either in the database or in the analysis data set which creates a complete date. Depending on the circumstances, the algorithm to create the full date can make some assumptions to fill in missing pieces. For example, if the day is missing, it might assign "1." Sometimes there is a fifth field that is associated with the set which indicates whether the date was full specified as collected or is based on an assumption or has the date stored as a text string in an alternate format. See Figure 3.1 for an illustration of this approach.

A study may well have dates that fall into all three categories. Discussions with biostatisticians on the types of analyses to be performed will clarify which dates must be complete, which can be stored as partial dates for reference, and which can be approximated to allow some information to be extracted from them. Some database designers will mix and match date-field

CRF:Adverse event start date: __/__/____ (month, day, year)

Database fields: AE_START_MM defined as 2 characters
AE_START_DD defined as 2 characters
AE_START_YYYY defined as 4 characters
AE_START_DATE defined as a date but derived
DATE_STATUS defined as a character but derived

Derivations:

AE_START_DATE would be the combination of date parts converted to a date data type if all three pieces were present. Depending on the meaning of the field, one option would be to fill in "01" if the day were missing and even to fill in "06" (for June) if the month were missing. The value would be left empty if the year were missing.

DATE_STATUS might be derived to a value of "Y" if all three parts are present, to "N" if day or month is missing, and to "D" (for discrepancy) if the year is missing.

Examples:

Reported Date	AE_START_MM	AE_START_DD	AE_START_YYYY	AE_START_DATE	DATE_COMPLETE
06/12/1998	06	12	1998	06/12/1998	Y
06/ /1998	06		1998	06/01/1998	N
/ /1998				(empty)	D

Figure 3.1 An illustration of using a set of fields to avoid problems in collecting and storing incomplete dates.

approaches while others will opt for a single multifield approach and use it for all date fields to assure consistency for entry and reporting.

Text fields and annotations

Clinical data from any of the common sources, such as CRFs, electronic entry screens, and electronic files, always contain some text. The most common text-type fields are:

- Categorical (coded) values
- Short comments
- Reported terms
- Long comments
- Annotations on the page

All of these text-data types require special handling, especially so when the text data is to be analyzed and not just used for medical review or safety monitoring.

Coded values

Categories of answers, often known as coded values, comprise the largest number of text fields. These fields have a limited list of possible answers and usually can contain only those answers. Common examples of coded fields include "Yes/No" answers, "Male/Female" for gender, and "Mild/ Moderate/Severe" for severity. The list of possible answers is usually known as a "codelist" and contains a short code that is stored as well as a longer value that corresponds to the data capture instrument.

Coded text fields only present a problem if the associated field can contain more than one answer or if the answer frequently falls outside the predefined list. When more than one answer is possible, the database design changes from a single field with a single answer to a series of fields, each of which may hold any eligible response from the codelist. See Figure 3.2 for an example. If the answer is frequently not in the predefined list, a coded value may not be appropriate, or a value of "Other" may be needed. If there is a category "Other" in a codelist, there frequently is a related field on the collection form defined as: "If other, specify." The value provided in this field is usually a short free text, though it may be another coded field that provides access to a larger, more comprehensive, list of categories.

Short texts

A very common short-comment field is that associated with a "Normal/ Abnormal" response labeled "If abnormal, explain." Medical-history terms or "Reason for Discontinuation" fields are other common examples of short text. These responses can be reviewed for clinical or safety

CRF page:
　Treatment required (check one):　[ ] None　[ ] OTC　[ ] Prescription Drug　[ ] Hospitalization
　　　　　　　　　　　　　　　　　[ ] Nondrug Therapy
Database design:　　　　　　　　　TRT_REQ defined as a coded numeric field
　　　　　　　　　　　　　　　　　TREATMENT codelist defined with the
possible values:
1 NONE
2 OTC
3 PRESCRIPTION
4 HOSPITALIZATION
5 NON_DRUG_THERAPY
CRF page:
　Treatment required (check all that apply):　　[ ] None　[ ] OTC　[ ]
Prescription Drug
　　　　　　[ ] Hospitalization　　[ ] Nondrug Therapy
Database design #1:　TRT_NONE defined as a coded field with YES/NO
　　　　　　　　　　TRT_OTC defined as a coded field with YES/NO
　　　　　　　　　　TRT_PRESCRIPTION defined as a coded field with YES/NO
　　　　　　　　　　TRT_HOSPITAL defined as a coded field with YES/NO
　　　　　　　　　　TRT_NON_DRUG defined as a coded field with YES/NO
Database design #2:　TREATMENT defined as a text field; entry staff enter a string
　　　　　　　　　　of comma-separated numbers, such as "2, 3".

Figure 3.2 An example of a database design for a coded field with a single answer versus a design for a field with multiple answers. The example refers to a treatment-required field typically found on AE CRF pages.

monitoring, but it is difficult to analyze them because any kind of summarization or analysis of these values depends on some consistency of the data.

Unfortunately, with many of these short and important texts, codelists are not practical as the groupings are not apparent until analysis takes place. The best that can be done for those is to standardize spelling, spacing, and symbols as much as possible.

Reported terms

If the short texts or comments are important to the study, a codelist, possibly a very large one, should be used to group like texts. Large codelists (sometimes called dictionaries or thesauri) are available for a very common class of short free-text fields: AEs, medications, and diagnoses. These kinds of free text are often called reported terms and the matching of the terms to a codelist is a complex coding process. (See the coding section of Chapter 9 for more information on coding reported terms, and Chapter 23 for more information on the large codelists.)

Long texts

Longer texts, those that cover several lines, are usually associated with a group of fields or even an entire page or visit. Clinical research associates and medical monitors use this text to cross-check against other problems reported or found in the data. Long texts are never analyzed.

The length of the text can pose serious problems for the database designer because some databases, query tools, and analysis programs have limitations on the length of text fields to which easy access is provided. (That is, very long comments take more work to extract.) Long comments can be stored in several ways:

- As one large text field
- As several numbered text fields
- In a separate storage area
- In CRF images only, with a cross reference in the data

Some database systems can store texts several thousand characters long. In this case, a single field is likely to meet the needs of the long comment and has the advantage of making data entry and review straightforward. However, many reporting applications still have limits on the text that are in the hundreds of characters. So, even if the database application does not impose limits, the query tool may not be able to extract the full text, or the analysis tool may not be able to include the field without truncation. Because of this, options other than a single field frequently must be considered.

One common solution is to store the text in a series of numbered short fields grouped with the other related fields (i.e., in the same database record)

(Figure 3.3). A series of related text fields has several drawbacks. The designer must guess the number of fields to create, and data entry staff must determine the best way of breaking up the text between lines. Also, review of the complete long text requires the extraction and reformatting of the entire set of fields, which usually makes ad hoc retrievals of the text impractical.

Some database designers get around the inconvenience of numbered fields by storing the comments separately in their own data structure or grouping them using the tall-skinny database format (described later in this chapter). In this approach, shown in Figure 3.4, the grouping (database record) consists only of the needed header and identifying information and a single-comment field of appropriate width. When more room is needed for the comments, they are entered in additional rows of the grouping. With this structure, there is no need to guess at the maximum number of fields

CRF page: Comment on any abnormal findings:

Database design: COMMENT_L1 defined as a 60-character text
COMMENT_L2 defined as a 60-character text
COMMENT_L3 defined as a 60-character text
COMMENT_L4 defined as a 60-character text

All appearing in the same database record.

Patient ID	Visit	. . .	COMMENT_L1	COMMENT_L2	COMMENT_L3	COMMENT_L4

Figure 3.3. Storing long comment text in a series of short, numbered fields.

CRF page: Comment on any abnormal findings:

Database design: appropriate header information

COMMENT defined as a 60-character text.

Patient ID	Visit	Page	LINE_NO	COMMENT

Data storage would look like:

Patient ID	Visit	Page	LINE_NO	COMMENT
1001	2	24	1	This is the first line of a long comment.
1001	2	24	2	This is the second line of a long comment.
1001	2	24	3	This is the third line of a long comment.

Figure 3.4 Example of using a "tall-skinny" data structure to store long comments.

or size of the text, but the data entry staff is still faced with the question of how to separate the lines of text. Ad hoc reporting from a column of comments is a bit easier than from a series of fields, but care must be taken if the database application does not automatically keep internal information on the order of lines. Also, if the comments are regularly reviewed along with the rest of the data then a query will have to reference two storage locations and join the data together appropriately.

Storage of texts

With long and short text fields, and in fact with any field, there is little point in adjusting the size of the field to minimize overall database size. Disk space does not present a problem with today's technology, even for the largest studies. Hard disks and backup media are not expensive compared to the other costs of the study, and most database applications only use as much space as is needed by the data — that is, the individual database records are not expanded to their maximum possible width based on the record design. The data takes up only as much space as it needs plus some record overhead. Database designers should make a good guess based on known studies and leave plenty of space for integers and text.

Header information

To identify where a given set of data comes from, patient information such as investigator, patient number, and patient initials always appears with it when it is collected. Usually there is also a visit indicator and/or visit date to identify the time point in the study at which the data was collected. On paper CRFs, this information is found in a header box at the top of each page. On electronic CRFs, it appears on each screen. In electronic files of lab data, the header information may be found once in the file, once in a section, or on every line. Requiring the repetition of patient or other header information during collection helps ensure that the assignment of any given data to the patient is correct.

Patient-header information is common to all trials, but there are other fields that may be needed to identify the data and its place in the study or may be required for specific data management applications or systems. Examples of such other header fields include:

- Page number
- Page type or name (e.g., AE, DEMOG, PHYSEX)
- Document identifier

On storing this data in a database, good database-design theory would call for techniques to assure that the header information be stored only once and then be related to all the remaining data through one or more key codes. (Only the key code is then stored with each grouping or record of data.) Good theory and technique, however, may not always be practical for data management where we often choose to copy header information to each grouping or record.

Facilitating the cleaning of the data is one of the best and most practical reasons for deviating from the store only once rule. For example, if CRF pages are received singly from a site or can be separated, it can be a very good policy to enter the patient-header information new for each page and run discrepancy checks against initial enrollment information. This would ensure that the header data was transcribed to the CRF properly and then entered in the database with the correct association. If dates vary within a single visit, that information should be captured and appropriately associated with each set of data, as it may affect analysis. This might mean storing the date more than once per visit. Duplicating values may also be necessary to other systems integrated with, or dependent on, the data management database, such as when a document ID must be stored with each record or piece of data to allow automatic connections from the data to an imaging system version of the CRF.

Some clinical data management (CDM) systems allow the designer to make the decision of whether or not to duplicate the header information or store it only once. Other systems store the patient identifiers only once and allow the designer to decide for the remaining header information. Still other systems enforce the idea of not duplicating data. No matter which approach a company must use or chooses to use, data management must be aware of the implications and set up a process to identify and correct problems with header information.

Single check boxes

In good CRF design, questions do not have "blank" as an acceptable answer, since blanks may be confused with overlooked fields or unavailable answers. The blank answer occurs most commonly with single answer check boxes such as:

Check if any adverse events: [ ]

If the box is checked, the answer is that, yes, there are AEs. If the box is blank, then either there are no AEs or the field was overlooked. (See Chapter 2 for further discussion on this topic.) Because data managers, especially at contract research organizations (CROs), do not always have a say in the design of CRF pages, they may be faced with designing a database to support these types of fields.

All the options for a database design to support single check boxes store the information of whether or not the box was checked, but they have different philosophical angles:

- Associate a Yes/No codelist with the field
- Associate a Yes-only codelist with the field
- Do not use a codelist

When a Yes/No codelist is associated with a single-check type of field, some companies have data entry enter "No" when the field is blank. Entering "No" does not truly reflect what is on the CRF and so may be contrary to company guidelines on entering exactly what is seen. Other companies using "Yes/No" codelists have data entry use the blank value — never actually entering "No." This can introduce problems if "No" can still be entered. The association of the field to the codelist has the potential of introducing confusion as it seems to imply that more responses are possible than the CRF would permit.

Using a codelist containing "Yes" only, or some other value that means "checked," gets around the potential confusion of using a Yes/No codelist because it clearly limits the possible responses. It does introduce the need for yet another codelist that does little more than ensure consistency at entry. Since a Yes-only codelist offers little in the way of categorizing responses, some companies just use a single character to indicate that a box or field was checked. This may be an "X," a "Y," or even a "1." These groups then typically include additional discrepancy checking at, or after, entry to catch inappropriate values.

Calculated or derived values

Data from the CRF, electronic entry screens, and electronic files are not the only data associated with a study. There are internal fields that can be convenient and even very important to the processing of data that are calculated from other data using mathematical expressions or are derived from other data using text algorithms or other logic. Examples of calculated values include age (if date of birth is collected), number of days on treatment (when collecting treatment dates), weight in kilograms (if it is collected in pounds) or standard international (SI) lab values (when a variety of lab units are collected). Examples of derived values include extracting site identifier from a long patient identifier, assigning a value to indicate whether a date was complete (see above), and matching dictionary codes to reported AE terms. Some of these values are calculated or derived in analysis data sets; others are calculated or derived in the central database.

Database designers should identify the necessary calculated and derived fields and determine whether they will be assigned values as part of analysis or as part of the central database. If the values for internal fields are needed for discrepancy identification or report creation, then storing them in the database may be the most sensible approach. If the values are used only during analysis, there may be no need to create permanent storage for them. Note that calculating or deriving values in the database means that the expression or algorithm is written only once and run consistently, whereas when calculations are performed at the time of analysis, the algorithm may have to be duplicated in several locations. In this case, filling the derived values centrally reduces the effort to write, validate, and run the calculation or derivation.

Special integers

Patient-identifier fields look perfectly benign and numeric. However, a patient number represents a kind of numeric field that frequently causes problems because of the way the data is displayed. When the patient-number field is defined as an integer field, but the values are very long, many database and analysis systems will display the number in scientific notation. That is, a patient number such as 110001999 may display as "1.1e8." Even though the storage is correct, this is not a useful way to display patient identifiers. Other examples of fields prone to this problem include document IDs and batch numbers.

Patient-number fields may also have a leading zero problem. That is, a patient number may be "010004" for a site "01" and patient "0004." In most systems, leading zeros are stripped from numeric fields so that the value will appear as "10004." While this does not invalidate the value, it would be inconsistent with values on paper or in other systems.

To avoid either of these problems, define these special integer fields as text fields.

Tall-skinny versus short-fat

Our discussion of database designs up to this point has stayed away from the underlying structure of tables or records because many of the problems that clinical data fields present impact all applications. One design discussion that does require recognition of the underlying application is the discussion of "normalization" of a database. Database normalization, in general, is the process of creating a design that allows for efficient access and storage. More specifically, it usually involves a series of steps to avoid duplication or repetition of data by reducing the size of data groupings or records.

In some systems, database records are intrinsically linked to the CRF page so that choices regarding normalization are not available to the designer; in other systems, a high level of normalization is enforced and the designer has no say. In many CDM applications, the database designer may choose how much to normalize a design. This discussion is geared at making those choices.

Figure 3.5 shows an example of vital signs data stored in a non-normalized form and then the same data stored in one type of normalized form. (There are several levels of normalized forms that are not discussed here.) The normalized version of the table has fewer columns and more rows. The visual impact that normalization has on a table has led to the colloquial, easily remembered nicknames for these structures: short-fat for non-normalized tables and tall-skinny for the normalized form.

Both kinds of structures store the data accurately and allow for its appropriate retrieval, yet the choice impacts data management and analysis in several different ways. For example, data cleaning checks that compare start and end values of blood pressure at a single visit are much more easily performed in the short-fat format. Missing values are also more

Data storage in a short-fat form:

Patient ID	Visit	BP_DIA_1	BP_SYS_1	BP_DIA_2	BP_SYS_2	BP_DIA_3	BP_SYS_3
1001	2	120	72	118	70	117	68

Data storage in an example of a tall-skinny form:

Patient ID	Visit	Measure-ment	BP_DIA	BP_SYS
1001	2	1	120	72
1001	2	2	118	70
1001	2	3	117	68

Figure 3.5 An example of vital signs data stored in a non-normalized (short-fat) form and the same data stored in one normalized (tall-skinny) form.

easily detected in the short-fat form unless the entry and storage application assures that a row exists even when values are blank. Creation of the structures themselves and the associated checks is easier in the tall-skinny form since there are fewer fields and they are unique. Data querying is also easier in the tall-skinny form, since the field names containing data is clear and there is only one column per kind of field. The tall-skinny format does duplicate header data or other key data to each row. Unless the underlying entry application manages automatic propagation of changes to header information, it would be necessary to make updates individually in each and every row!

Clinical data contains many examples of repeated measurements that lend themselves well to storage in tall-skinny tables. These include physical exam (with columns for examination, normal/abnormal, and explanation if abnormal), medical history, x-rays (site, measurements), tumor assessments (site, description, size), AEs (event plus assessment), concomitant medications (name, route, dosage, frequency), and so on. In general, any data collected in a tabular format is a candidate for storing in tall-skinny form. Lists of related questions, each of which has the same kind of response, may also be stored this way if convenient. Inclusion and exclusion criteria are examples of this kind of list, with each question having the same Yes/No response (as long as there are no measurements tucked in among the questions).

In all of the examples above, the data in each column of the table is of the same kind and type. That is, a column contains data from a single kind of measurement. A data cleaning check, such as a range, applied to the column makes sense for each value in that column. The tall-skinny form is so flexible that it is sometimes applied to data where the values in a single column are not the same kind of measurement. Laboratory data is the classic example of this use of the tall-skinny form. One column may give the test name, one the test result, another the test units, and so on. (Note that a range applied to the test result would not be sensible as the values represent a variety of measurements.) See Chapter 8 for further discussion of using tall-skinny structures for this type of data.

Taking this idea of a tall-skinny table a few steps further, we can reach a point where a table contains the names of all the fields to be measured, their value, and other information related to the measurement. The additional information may include status of the data, such as whether the value has a discrepancy associated with it, whether it has been monitored at the site, and so on. This structure is sometimes called "hyper-normalized" and is the basis of some of the newer homegrown and vendor-developed CDM systems. Features and tools to conveniently access the data and also to reconfigure it for analysis are critical to these systems.

Using standards

Most companies have some standards in place for use in the design of a database and associated data entry screens. Standards simplify the process of designing and building database applications and also speed the process. Designers should be required to use existing fields, codelists, modules, tables, and other database objects within reason as obviously it is wrong to force a value into a field that does not truly reflect the content of the field and intent of the value. Yet, without strong requirements to use what is there (and sometimes even with those requirements), human nature and the desire to work fast always cause a proliferation of database fields that are really the same but are defined with different names and slightly varying characteristics. Besides causing more work at the time of creation of the database, they greatly increase the effort required for validation of the database application and also of the analysis programs.

Applications vary widely in how they support and enforce standard attributes of database objects. Some, such as systems linked tightly to CRF pages, may not have checks on standards at all. Others, such as large applications that support a range of data management activities, may support different levels of standards enforcement that must be set or turned on after installation or even on a study basis. In all cases, a process supporting the technology should be in place to avoid undue proliferation of items. The process for using standards should define and manage:

- New fields
- Variations on fields
- New codelists
- Additions to codelists
- Changes in groups of fields

and all other additions to, or deviations from, previous database designs.

Larger firms may have a standards committee or a standards czar who reviews all new items and enforces standards with special tools. The committee or czar may be the only ones empowered to define new objects and sometimes they are the only ones with permission to actually create those objects in the application. These committees have value in that they create a person or group that has good oversight over both the philosophy of database design and the particulars of the database objects used by all projects. Unfortunately, they can become unwieldy and delay work by not meeting frequently enough, by taking too long to produce a new object, and by not providing enough people with privileges to create objects (thereby causing difficulties when someone is out).

Even small data management groups will benefit from having one or two people who review database designs so that the philosophy is similar and the fields are defined consistently. Even a little bit of standardization can go a long way to reducing setup time and the associated validation of the database application.

In all companies, true standards can only be achieved when the CRF or eCRF module is standardized as well. The most successful standardization efforts involve clinical teams, programmers, and statisticians working with data management and within database systems restrictions. Standardization effort will not work unless all department managers commit to following the standards that are developed!

After deciding on a design

Deciding on a design is just the first step in creating a database, and the most time-consuming. The design is documented to form a specification that guides the actual database-building process. At a minimum, an annotated CRF is used to document the design, but companies may also require a separate design document. Chapter 4 discusses the specification, testing, and building of the database or EDC application in detail.

Quality assurance for database design

Use of standards and reuse of similar modules are the best ways to ensure quality in database design. Every time a new database object is used and put into production, it opens up a chance for design errors. Even when standard objects are used for new studies, the designer may choose the wrong object. Database design is a critical step in conducting a study and a policy of "do and review" should be in place. That is, one person does the work and another reviews it.

Review is important here because a poor database design may adversely impact not only entry but also data cleaning, extraction or listing programs, and analysis. Something as simple as a missing field in the database can impact production timelines as CRFs stack up for paper studies or a new version of an EDC application must be released. Just as programmers on critical applications in other industries have software code review, database designs should always be reviewed by a second person. Even the smallest of data management groups should be able to arrange for some level of review as it is not practical or wise to have only one person able to do a particular task.

Standard operating procedures for database design

The procedures guiding database designs are frequently included as part of the database creation or setup standard operating procedures (SOPs). If there is a separate SOP on design, it might discuss the use of standards and the process for requesting new kinds of database objects. Such an SOP should require as output from the design process an annotated CRF and possibly a database design document.

Responsibilities in database design

As CDM systems become both more sophisticated and at the same time easier to use, more data managers are becoming involved in the design and creation of the central databases and entry applications. This is both appropriate and efficient. Data managers know the typical data closely and are often aware of the problems associated with a particular collection method. With training in the application, a little background on the issues, and a good set of standards from which to build, database design or database building can be an interesting addition to the tasks of experienced data managers.

Development of EDC systems is, as of today, performed by programmers. Because data managers are much more familiar with the characteristics of the data than a typical programmer, they are a critical component to the design of entry screens and underlying database objects for these systems. As we will see in the next chapter, they are likely to be involved in user acceptance testing for these systems if they are not, themselves, building the database.

chapter four

Study setup

Building a database and preparing a study for production entry of data is building an application. It may not look like programming, but using an application is just like using a high-level programming language, even if there is no "if-then-else" in sight. Because the database application will be used to create records of clinical data, and that data is the basis of decisions on the safety and efficacy of the treatment, and because the data may be used to support a submission to the Food and Drug Administration, a database application for a study falls under Good Clinical Practice (GCP) guidelines and 21 CFR 11 requirements for validation. The Society for Clinical Data Managers (SCDM) also makes a point of this approach in the "Database Validation, Programming and Standards" chapter of their Good Clinical Data Management Practices document.

As we will see in detail in Chapter 20, validation is more than testing. Roughly speaking, validation requires a plan, a specification of what is to be built, testing after it is built, and change control once it is in production use. In the case of building and releasing a database application for a study:

- A standard operating procedure (SOP) acts as the validation plan
- The annotated case report form (CRF) plus design document is the specification
- The final database design and associated entry screens are tested with typical data
- A change control system is put into place as production data is being entered

In this chapter, we discuss each of these bullet points in more detail, focusing on the process for setting up a classic clinical data management (CDM) database to collect data from paper CRFs. The same concepts also apply to electronic data capture (EDC) systems, but ideas specific to those applications will be addressed as they arise. The discussion of edit checks (data validation) is specifically not discussed in this chapter; see Chapter 7 for information on building and releasing edit check programs.

35

A plan for validation

If you do not have a plan, you will not know what to do to declare an application as "validated." For study setup in a CDM system, a data management SOP that describes the steps necessary to build, test, release, and maintain a database application for a study can act as the validation plan for all studies. The validation plan in the form of an SOP will detail all the steps necessary to build and release a system and keep it in a validated state. The high-level steps are explained in more detail below. For each step, the SOP should also describe what kind of output is to be produced as evidence that the step was carried out. Typically, that output would be filed in the study file or binder (see Chapter 1).

Specification and building

In Chapter 3, the concept of designing a database before building it was introduced. The output from the design process for a given study is a specification of the database that is to be built. The specification is, at a minimum, an annotated CRF. Quite a few companies require a database design document in addition to the annotated CRF.

For CDM, the annotated CRF is usually a blank CRF that has written on it (by hand or as an electronic overlay) the names of the database column, field, or item associated with each CRF field. The CRF page is also clearly marked to show how questions are grouped into modules or tables. Because the annotated CRF is used not only by the database designer but also by edit check writers, entry screen designers, and even those browsing data through database queries, it is helpful if the codelists associated with an item are present along with any hidden, internal, or derived fields associated with each module (see descriptions in Chapter 3). The use of annotated CRFs is widespread enough to be considered industry standard practice.

A separate design document, while not required by all data management groups, can provide information that is not readily obvious from the annotated CRF. This document might include simple overview information such as the list of all groupings or tables and the names of all codelists used. In companies where there are firm CRF page and database standards, the design document can focus on deviations from those standards (if any) and introduce any new objects created for this study. It might also include a more detailed discussion of design decisions that were made for problematic fields or tables.

The database builder uses these specifications to create the database objects for a study. The building process itself acts as another form of database review. The designer may notice a problem with the design or may not be able to implement the object as specified. The designer and builder then work to find a solution and update the specification documents appropriately. Typically, the builder will work in a development environment that mimics the actual production environment, that is, the base software versions and standard objects are the same but development work is taking place "on the side." When the application is ready for testing, that testing may take place in the development environment, yet another area specifically set up for testing, or in the production environment itself.

Testing

Validation always involves testing as one element of the process and all clinical database applications should be tested, without exception! A mistake in the creation of the database or a poor design choice will impact data storage and possibly analysis. Testing aims to identify these errors before production data is stored in the application so that changes can be made without impacting live data. Just as with software testing, one has to take a practical approach and decide what kind and what amount of testing is most likely to identify problems, without taking up too many resources and too much time.

The testing of a clinical database application most naturally takes place when the entry screens are ready using patient test data written on CRFs. Depending on the complexity of the study, data management groups will typically test the data from 2 to 10 patients. If the goal is purely to test the entry screens, the test data will be mostly normal data with typical exceptions in date formats or text in numeric fields. Some companies use data that will later be used to test edit checks as test data, in which case many values will be chosen to later fail the edit checks.

Ideally, data entry staff will perform the entry of the test data as if it were real. Any problems that they identify in the fields or in the flow of the screens should lead to corrections and an appropriate level of re-entry of the test data. But the testing should not stop once data entry is flowing smoothly!

After the data has been entered, the responsible data manager should run the process or programs to fill in any derived or calculated fields. Then a tester should compare data extracted from the database against the original test CRFs as if this were a data audit. Besides looking to see if the data values match, the tester is also checking:

- Is the data stored in the correct field?
- Are the calculated variables calculated and correct?
- Are all hidden variables filled in as needed?
- Has any data been truncated or otherwise improperly stored?
- Are there unexpected blank records?
- Are fields that should be carried over to multiple rows or groups properly carried?

There may also be additional checks that are related to the application used to capture the data. This step of comparing the extracted data to the original is often overlooked but should not be. Finding any of the above problems is a very serious situation and it may be impossible to correct once data is in production.

Since a validation process requires documentation of each step, the test data and results should be filed in the study file as evidence of the process. Many companies also print a report of the final database structure along with screens, if warranted by the application they are using. The study is now almost ready to move into production use.

Moving to production

We know that validation is not just testing. Therefore, completing the testing does not mean that validation is complete. There are usually several additional steps necessary before production entry and processing can begin. At the very least, study specific training must take place before live data is entered.

Entry staff should be trained on the new study. This training is not a complex formal training on the application and company standards; rather, it focuses on study specific issues. Typical preproduction entry training will include a discussion of difficult or nonstandard entry screens and a review of standard and study specific data entry conventions or guidelines. Evidence of the training should be filed in the study file or in each employee's training binder. Frequently, a CDM group will also require a record of signatures and initials in the study file for anyone who will work on the study. This is a good point to collect the initial set. After training, and only after training, should entry staff be given access or permissions on the data in the new production study. (For more on training, see Chapter 13.)

In addition to training, it is quite common to have additional requirements that must be met before production use of a study application. These may include, for example:

- Sign-off by biostatistics on the database design
- Setup of related tracking and reporting applications for the new study
- Moving of the application into a production area

When there are many steps involved in releasing a study for entry, it is always worth having a checklist so that no step is ever overlooked. Even if the checklist is not a controlled document or required as part of an SOP, it provides value to the people doing the work and improves quality because critical steps will not be missed.

Change control

During the course of carrying out a study, it is very likely that a change to the database design will be needed. The change may be due to unexpected data coming in from the site (such as texts longer than originally anticipated), texts are showing up where only numeric values were expected, or perhaps the protocol has been amended and now requires that additional data be collected during a visit. After carefully validating the application, a change made willy-nilly can result in putting the database application in an unvalidated state.

Once a system has been validated, it will only stay validated if no changes are made to the application. Larger software systems, such as the database systems, are under change control once they have been validated. Changes are carefully tracked and appropriate testing and documentation is required. The same should apply to database applications for individual studies. In the case of a database application for a study, it is important to consider what a change to the database application *is* and what *is not* a change. Adding, deleting, or modifying patient data according to standard practices and under audit trail is not a change to the application and does require change control. In most systems, adding users and granting access (again, using appropriate procedures) is not a change to the system. Adding fields, lengthening text fields, and modifying entry screens are all examples of changes that should be carried out under a change control process.

A change control process can be quite simple. It requires that responsible staff members:

- Define what the change is and how it will be made
- Get review or approval for the change prior to making it
- Assess the impact of the change on the application, the data, and training
- Show evidence of appropriate testing

If a sophisticated change control system is not available, this information can be recorded on paper and stored in a change control binder, or it can be entered into a simple log file or spreadsheet. Many of the most common changes can be documented and carried out with a few sentences in the log or on the form. However, more complex changes that have several interlinked requirements or those that impact several groups would benefit from having a targeted document, in addition to a simple change control log entry, to describe the change process and impact in detail.

Some examples will help clarify the requirements. The case of lengthening a text field provides us with an example of a low-impact change. Existing data is unlikely to be affected. The database definition will change but (depending on the system) the change may have no impact on entry screens. It is worth considering whether edit checks, listings, and so forth are affected by the greater length text, but if the answer is "no," then a simple log entry with this information in the impact-assessment field would be sufficient.

Now consider the example of adding a field to the database because a protocol amendment requires that the sites now record the time a certain procedure is performed. Adding a field is an example of a change that might have broad impact. In addition to the actual database change, adding a field touches on:

- The annotated CRF
- The CRF or eCRF completion guidelines
- One or more entry screens
- Data management instructions on what to do if the old form comes in with no time field
- Edit specifications and the associated cleaning rules
- Possibly data transfer programs
- Possibly listings or other reports

If this is in an EDC system, the change would impact all sites, so notification, if not training, would be required. This case shows us that if multiple areas or users are affected, or any impact cannot be described in one or two sentences, then a more detailed change plan is warranted.

Setup for EDC systems

Development of EDC applications for a study follows similar requirements for validation. However, because so much more is built into an EDC application as an integral part of the system, the specification step is more complex and takes longer. The specification document may not be an annotated CRF but it may be the protocol plus any other study specific requirements for the screens or even mockups of screens. It may also include many of the edit checks that are programmed separately in traditional systems, and the specification frequently includes the structure of transfer datasets. The fact that all these things are programmed into the application, often by a separate EDC programming group, is the main reason that data management groups should allot a larger block of time for study setup and building for EDC studies than for paper based studies.

While experienced data managers are able to set up studies in the more traditional data management systems, it is currently the case that EDC applications are programmed by programming groups. These groups will take the specifications and work with the "client" data management team to build the application. Typically, they will perform the initial system and/or validation testing, but then data management will carry out additional testing, usually called "user acceptance testing," that determines if the EDC application not only works but also meets the needs of the study as they see it.

Change control is even more critical in an EDC system because changes impact the sites directly. Because of the serious impact that even minor changes will have on an EDC application and its users, a more formal version control or release system is appropriate. These version control or release systems are, or are like, those that a software company would use.

Quality assurance

Care in building and releasing a database cannot be stressed enough. Because even the best and most experienced designers and builders make mistakes, those responsible for setting up a database should implement a policy of "do and review." Chapter 3 recommended that a reviewer go over the database design before building starts. Building the database from specifications is another form of review. Then, after building is complete, we have data entry and the data comparison testers who are reviewing the data from the database build. In all of these steps, the review is not a policing action where the reviewer is looking to catch the first person making a mistake; rather, it is a collaborative effort to identify potential problems.

As we will see in Chapter 5, many groups find that errors are introduced not during initial entry but when values need to be edited later. Similarly, many companies have a solid process for releasing databases but introduce errors when they make changes. Looking more closely at change control can improve quality of the process and the data.

SOPs for study setup

In order to avoid writing a validation plan for each study database setup, an SOP needs to be in place that will be general enough to suit all studies and yet specific enough to satisfy the requirements for validation. Change control may be part of that study database setup SOP or it may be discussed in detail in another procedure. The actual checklist for moving a study into production may or may not be part of the SOPs, but the requirement to have a checklist may be explicitly called for.

Setup is programming

In today's EDC systems, it is still clear that study setup is a programming task. In the traditional data management systems, the setup process may not appear to be programming since it is performed through user interfaces; and yet it is programming. In fact, it is programming that has a huge impact on the data that is to be collected from a clinical trial. For that reason, every database setup should be validated as an application that will affect safety and efficacy decisions for the treatment in question.

chapter five

Entering data

When data for a clinical study is captured on paper case report forms (CRFs), that data must be transferred to a database for final storage. We will call the process of transferring it from paper or image into electronic storage "data entry." Data entry may be entirely manual or it may be partly computerized using optical character recognition (OCR). Regardless of whether there is a computerized step involved in the process, and regardless of the specific application used, the main data entry issues that must be addressed by technology or process, or both, are:

- Selecting a method to transcribe the data
- Determining how closely data must match the CRF
- Creating processes to deal with problem data
- Making edits and changing data without jeopardizing quality
- Quality control of the entire process

Transcribing the data

Accurately transcribing the data from the CRF to the database is essential. Errors in transcription are usually due to typographical errors ("typos") or illegibility of the values on the CRF. Companies aim to reduce transcription errors using one of these methods:

- Double data entry with third party reconciliation of discrepancies
- Double data entry with second person resolving discrepancies
- Single entry with extensive data checking
- OCR as first entry with one or more subsequent entry or review passes

Even after transcription errors are reduced to a minimum, there remains some variation in what an accurate transcription means. Does it mean that the data is an *exact* duplicate of the values found on the CRF, or are there deviations or variations permitted?

Double entry

With its error rate often given as .1 to .2%, double data entry has long been used without question as a reliable method of transcription. In double entry, one operator enters all the data in a first pass, and then an independent second operator enters the data again. Two different techniques are used to identify mismatches and also to resolve those mismatches.

In one double entry method, the two entries are made and both are stored. After both passes have been completed, a comparison program checks the entries and identifies any differences. Typically, a third person reviews the report of differences and makes a decision as to whether there is a clear correct answer (for example, because one entry had a typo) or whether a discrepancy must be registered because the data value is illegible or is in some other way unclear. This method of double entry is sometimes known as "blind" double entry since the operators have no knowledge of each other's work.

The other double entry method uses the second entry operator to resolve mismatches. After first pass entry, the second entry operator selects a set of data and begins to re-enter it. If the entry application detects a mismatch, it stops the second operator who decides, right then and there, what the correct value should be or whether to register a discrepancy to be resolved by a third person. This double entry method does not have a common name but will be referred to as "heads-up second entry."

Blind double entry is well suited to the use of temporary or untrained staff for both entry passes. A more experienced operator or coordinator is usually used to act as the third person reviewing the discrepancies identified by comparing the passes. Heads-up second entry works best if the second entry pass is performed by a more experienced operator, but many companies have seen good success with this method even when using temporary staff. If the entry application supports it, it would be worth considering using different methods at different times or with different studies, depending on available staff.

Extensive checks at entry time are rarely incorporated into entry applications when data is to be entered in two passes. A check at entry would only slow down the operators and would bring little value. Checks on the data is run after differences have been resolved.

Single entry

While relatively rare in traditional clinical data management, single entry is an option when there are strong supporting processes and technologies in place to identify possible typos or errors because of unclear data. Electronic data capture (EDC) is a perfect example of single-pass entry; the site is the entry operator transcribing from source documents, and checks in the application immediately identify potential errors.

Single-pass entry could be considered an option in a traditional data management system when there are extensive checking routines built into the data entry application and further checks that run after entry. The entry operator would have to be trained in the protocol and encouraged to view the entry process as a quality and review process rather than as a simple transcription process. To address the concerns that there is a higher error rate, companies using single-pass entry could consider a more extensive audit of the data than would be used for double entry.

OCR plus review

OCR is a technique whereby software attempts to read text in a document. OCR has been used for many years to successfully read preprinted header information. As the software has improved, it has also been used to identify handwritten numbers and marks in check boxes. However, success rates in reading handwritten free text are still rather poor. As more companies move toward imaging or fax-in of CRFs, the opportunity to use OCR as a first entry pass has increased. When used, OCR becomes the first data entry pass on numbers and check boxes and is followed by at least one other pass to verify those numeric values and fill texts or other fields that could not be read by the OCR engine.

The second-pass operator (after OCR) visually checks values read by the OCR engine and types in any text values that appear on the form. Sometimes the OCR engine will provide an indicator of how sure it is about reading each value to guide the operator to fields that need review. Because the visual verification is hard to enforce and because the operator may fill in a significant number of fields, there is a danger of introducing transcription errors. Companies generally address this by doing yet another pass and also by including extensive post-entry checks.

How close a match?

We have discussed methods to help ensure accurate transcription of the data from the CRF, but what is accurate? Does accurate mean that the data in the database exactly matches that written into the CRF field? Are data entry operators given some leeway to substitute texts, make assumptions, or change the data? These questions must be clearly defined by each and every data management group.

Some companies do subscribe to the entry philosophy that the data transcribed from the CRF must match the CRF to the highest possible degree. Their guidelines tell the entry operators: "Type it as you see it; if it cannot be stored in the field, issue a discrepancy." One of the few exceptions at these companies would be if the CRF field contains symbols such as "↑" for "increasing." These are considered acceptable substitutions and are predefined and standard across studies.

Some firms allow more flexibility in the transcription of text fields, and some also permit changes to values found in numeric or date fields. However, it should be noted that the current industry trend is away from most changes at the time of entry. The feeling seems to be that except for symbols, data should be entered as seen or left blank; any changes are made after entry during the cleaning process so that there is a record of the change and the reason for it in the audit trail.

That being said, there still may be some changes permitted at entry time in addition to replacing symbols. Permitted changes to texts might include:

- Using standard notations for common units (e.g., "g" for "grams")
- Abbreviating some texts to fit in fields (e.g., using "pat." to replace "patient")
- Correcting some misspellings in comments and reported terms

An example of a permitted change to a numeric field would be to instruct data entry staff to enter the midpoint when a range of values is entered in a single field. That is, they enter "5" when the CRF reads "0–10." A correction to a date may be permitted to the year for study dates when the year changes. For example, in a study started in November 1998, data entry may correct visit dates written as January 1998 to January 1999. (See chapter 7 for a more detailed discussion of "self evident corrections.")

An accurately transcribed value may be a wrong value. That is, the value written on the CRF may be obviously incorrect or simply missing. If checks at entry time have been built into the entry application, those checks should never prevent entry staff from entering what they see.

Dealing with problem data

No matter how well designed a CRF is, there will be occasional problems with values in fields. The problems may be due to confusion about a particular question or they may be due to the person filling it out. The most common problem is illegibility; another is notations or comments in the margins. Sometimes pre-entry review of the CRFs can help manage these and other problems (but this can cause process problems in exchange). Because companies deal with these data problems in different ways, each data management group must specify the correct processing for each problem in data entry guidelines.

Illegible fields

Illegible writing on the CRF always causes problems for data entry, data management staff, and clinical research associates (CRAs). Each data management group should consider the following questions when planning an approach to illegible fields:

- Can entry operators discuss the value with each other?
- How do entry operators indicate illegibility at second pass?
  - Leave the field blank?
  - Guess and flag the field?
  - Type special flagging characters (e.g., "###")?
- Should data managers make educated guesses based on a review of other pages?
- Can the CRA make a decision based on medical information?

Even when staff tries to appropriately identify values, some data is just illegible and will have to be sent to the investigator for clarification during the data cleaning process.

Notations in margins

Investigators will sometimes supply data that is not requested. This most frequently takes the form of comments running in the margins of a CRF page but may also take the form of unrequested, repeated measurements written in between fields. Some database applications can support annotations or extra measurements that are not requested, but many cannot. If site annotations are not supported, data management, together with the clinical team, must decide what is to be done:

- Can the information be stored in the database as a comment or annotation (but then it could not be listed or analyzed)?
- Can the comment be ignored?
- Should the site be asked to remove the comment to transcribe it somewhere appropriate?

Many data management groups do not store unexpected information at all, but since it can contain medical information, senior data managers and/or CRAs will review the extra comments and measurements to look for important safety information.

Pre-entry review

In the past, many companies had an experienced data manager conduct a pre-entry review of all CRF pages. The reviewer wrote in code values for categorical fields (if they were not pre-printed), dealt with problems in header information, replaced "UNK" with "ND," tried to clarify texts that might be difficult to read and so forth. The idea was to speed up entry by dealing with significant issues ahead of time. The problem is that extensive review and in-house annotation circumvents the independent double entry process and its proven value. Because entry staff would enter whatever the reviewer wrote, and not consider whether that was appropriate or not, it was "one person decides." Also, in cases where the reviewer's notes changed the data or made assumptions, there was no audit trail of that information.

Now some companies still do a pre-entry review but it is minimal and focuses on issues that will prevent entry. More and more is being left to the entry operators. The entry staff is trained to identify and flag problem data appropriately. Review by a data manager only happens for significant issues. This is a better use of resources in that more senior staff members work only on problems, not normal data. It also encourages data to be entered as seen with changes and reasons recorded in the audit trail.

The philosophy toward pre-entry review does not have to be all or nothing. It is possible and sensible to satisfy both the need for smoother entry and the concerns of going too far by selecting an approach appropriate to the staff and supporting applications. For example, if incomplete or incorrect header information would actually prevent entry of any data from the page, then a data coordinator might review the header information while logging pages into the tracking system. A CRA or data coordinator might also review specific, troublesome data such as medications or adverse events (AEs) and clarify only those. The rest of the discrepancies may be left to the data entry staff to register manually or to the computer to register automatically. The data coordinator or CRA then addresses the discrepancies only after the data has been entered.

Modifying data

Initial entry is not the only entry task performed by data management. Following initial entry there are edits or corrections to the data. The corrections may have been identified internally in data management, by the CRA, or through an external query to the investigator. Just as there is a process for entry, there should be a well-defined process for making these corrections to the data.

Corrections may be made by regular entry staff or only by more senior staff. Some firms allow any entry operator to make corrections; others require a more experienced data manager to make changes. Many data entry or data management applications support different access privileges to data in different states, but if systems support is unavailable, the procedures must be enforced by process.

Most data management systems do not have a second pass on changes. The industry has found that errors are often introduced when changes are made. Clearly, rerunning cleaning checks on these new values is essential and that is assumed. Many companies have also instituted a visual review of changes. This may be done through the entry screen, through a report, or through the audit trail. Again, if the system does not support it, data management groups must put into place a process that ensures the visual review always takes place.

Any changes after initial entry, made by any person, should be recorded in an audit trail. The Food and Drug Administration requires audit trails to record changes made to clinical data (21 CFR 11), and it should be possible to view this audit trail at any time. There are, however, differences in how the term audit trail is interpreted and implemented. Firms and data management applications vary as to when, or at what state of the data, audit trails are "turned on." Some may audit changes after first entry, others after second pass is complete, and still others not until postentry cleaning routines have run. The form the audit trail takes, and the information associated with each implementation, adds further variations to audit trails across systems.

Quality control through database audits

CRF pages represent data management's source or raw data. The quality and correctness of the database is determined by checking the database data against the CRF and associated correction forms.

Quality assurance (QA) is a process, and quality control (QC) is a check of the process. QA for data entry builds on good standards and procedures and appropriately configured data entry applications. The approach that assures quality data entry is documented in the data management plan. QC for data entry is usually a check of the accuracy of the entry performed by auditing the data stored in the central database against the CRF. This is usually referred to as "database audit."

Data management staff carries out database audits to fulfill the QC function. Ideally, the auditors are not people who participated in data entry for that study. (External quality assurance groups at some companies perform this task to ensure independence of review.) They identify the CRFs to be used, pull the appropriate copies and associated query forms, and compare those values against the ones stored in the central database. The result of the audit is usually given as a number of errors against the number of fields on the CRF or in the database.

To conduct an audit, there must be a plan for the audit that includes:

- What data will be sampled
- Definition of an acceptable error rate
- A plan for what to do if the error rate is unacceptable

If the plan is consistent across studies, it can be defined in a standard operating procedure (SOP). If the plan is study specific, it can be laid out in the data management plan or in a separate audit plan document.

After the audit, a summary should document the final count of fields, total number of errors, error rate, and any action taken.

Audit plan

The number most frequently used in selecting data for an audit is 10%. This is often supplemented by a 100% audit of safety fields such as those for AEs. Some companies also audit 100% of a selection of key efficacy fields. It is very important to note that a "10% audit" still does not tell us exactly what was or will be audited. Is this 10% of the patients, pages, or data? Ten percent of the patients may be easy to select but does not guarantee good coverage of investigator sites. Ten percent of CRFs is better as long as all pages are represented. Ten percent of the data by data set is a very good sample but can be hard to program and hard to select the pages associated with that data.

Many companies say that their acceptable error rate is 1% to 5% (one to five percent). However, articles regarding this topic maintain that data as well controlled as clinical trial data should have errors only in the range of 10 to 50 per 10,000. This translates into .1% to .5%. This latter figure also is in line with numbers for high quality double entry and should be a good and reasonable target for most organizations.

What is to be done if the rate is unacceptable as a result of the audit? If the audit is early in the data management process, it may be possible to improve upon the process or systems to improve the rate. If the audit is performed at the end of the study, it would be advisable to increase the number of fields audited to confirm the rate. Some companies immediately plan a 100% audit of all of the data. Other companies perform another 10% sample. Still others examine the result first and try to determine if any particular type of data or specific data modules are the source of the problem. They then conduct 100% audit of just that data.

Audit report

The audit report is essentially a cover memo to the actual audit listings. It lists the number of errors, the number of fields counted, the final error rate, and any action taken. True differences between the database and the CRF and query forms count as database errors. Counting these rarely presents a problem. Counting the number of fields is a much harder problem and can have a significant impact on the error rate.

If the audit listings that have the database data is in the form of tables, one might think that simply multiplying rows by columns gives a count of fields. While this value is a count of the number of fields you looked at, the number of fields entered is not the same. For example, header information may appear in each row but was only entered once. Other values may have been repeated or duplicated across rows but only entered once. Some values may have been prefilled in the entry screen and not actually entered. While taking the simple multiplication route will result in a "better" error rate (because the denominator is bigger), groups that really want to know what the error rate is should investigate how to get the number fields in a conservative way that actually reflects how the data came to be in the database.

Even when the error rate is acceptable, it may be possible to detect some identifiable source or sources of errors. Retraining of data entry staff or data managers is always a possibility. But, since mismatches of the CRF data to the database can have many sources, it is possible that the feedback from the audit may go back to groups outside of data management. These may include:

- Database and screen designers and builders
- CRF designers
- Investigator site staff
- Site monitors

Feedback to these groups provides one of the greatest benefits of audits!

Audit process

Many firms perform an audit at or right after the close of a study. However, there is value in conducting an audit earlier in the process, or, in fact, during the entire process. Small audits conducted throughout the study may identify problems with training staff at the site, problems at the sponsor in transcribing the data, or problems with the entry application. Since locking the study is usually a key time point with tight deadlines, doing some of the work earlier on may also improve the time to close.

Whenever an audit is conducted, the listings, with errors highlighted and any summary or review, should be filed in the study files.

SOPs for data entry

At companies with a very consistent entry process, the process itself may be laid out in an SOP. For example, a data entry SOP may always require blind double entry with third party arbitration of discrepancies. It may also indicate the level of pre-entry review and outline the audit process. At companies with variations in data entry across groups or studies, the SOP may only state a commitment to accuracy and indicate that local guidelines are to be followed and methods documented. The data management plan is a good place to identify any study specific exceptions or changes to the standard procedures.

Enter quality

As the saying goes: "Garbage in, garbage out." Data in the database is only as good as the collection method; so when data entry is used, it should be considered an essential step in assuring quality. Quality comes from using people and technology appropriately and efficiently. When using inexperienced or temporary help, encourage them to think quality rather than speed.

They are the first line of defense on identifying problems with the CRFs, the sites, the entry application, and sometimes the central database. When using technology, have it do what it is good at — this usually means checking the data and may also include initial entry through OCR. In general, don't duplicate manual tasks with system tasks; find a way to make better use of both and apply the resources where they provide the most benefit.

chapter six

Tracking CRF pages and corrections

When entry is performed from paper or images, companies need to track case reports forms (CRFs) through the data management process to assure that all the data makes it into the storage database. Some companies take tracking a step further and track the *data* from the CRF pages through the rest of the data management process, while keeping the connection between the data and the page from which it came. Keeping the connection through data cleaning, discrepancy resolution, analysis, and quality control can greatly improve the efficiency of those tasks.

Tracking can be performed successfully entirely on paper and by hand. Yet, the most useful tracking systems are those integrated with data management applications. The benefits of a good tracking system are surprisingly high and can result in a considerable reduction in the time spent on annoying administrative tasks associated with shuffling paper. They can also introduce a higher level of confidence in quality of processing.

Goals of tracking

The primary goal of any tracking method is to assure that data is not lost and this goal *must* be met. Companies may identify additional goals for their tracking systems. For example, they may want to quickly obtain information on the status of the data in the data management system: is it entered, has it had a second entry pass, or are there any outstanding discrepancies? Companies may also want to use the information in tracking systems as input into planning for future studies by making available metrics on required resources, elapsed time, and effort for processing completed studies. Both the required and secondary goals are met by knowing where the CRF pages (paper or image) are in the entry part of the process.

To meet the primary goal, data management staff uses tracking information to know which CRFs have been received by the group and whether the data from those CRFs has been entered. Reports or summaries of expected but missing pages help identify any CRFs that might have been misplaced or overlooked (more on this below). Separate tracking of data updates via query forms ensures that the data has actually been updated, if required. The more advanced goals of tracking systems are best met by following the data from the pages through the rest of the data management cycle while keeping a reference to the source page intact.

CRF workflow

Do you know where your pages are? Tracking a CRF, paper or image, involves knowing where the page is in the data management process. The path the pages follow and the stops they make (or states they are in) is often known as the workflow. Some workflow states common to most data management processes are:

- Received by data management
- Entry — first pass or initial optical character recognition
- Entry — second pass
- Discrepancies outstanding
- Completed and filed

Other states would be application- or process-dependent and may include such information as: have some or all cleaning checks been run over the data, has the data been transferred out (e.g., from a contract research organization (CRO) to a client or from data management to biostatistics), and has the data has been audited against the page.

In paper tracking systems or simple computerized systems (e.g., using an Excel spreadsheet), when a page goes to a new stop in the workflow, its state must be updated manually. More sophisticated or integrated systems can generally update more, but generally not all, of the states automatically. For example, a more integrated system may require that a page be logged in manually as "received" but then be able to update the state of the page to "entered" and "second entered" automatically.

Balancing the desire to know the exact status of a page with the effort to determine that status is a challenge to all tracking systems. If a group needs to know that a page has been received independent of whether it has been entered (and imaging is not being used), then a manual update of state is necessary. Another group may feel that first entry is sufficient evidence that a page has been received and may choose to avoid the manual logging step. While updating one or two states manually is not uncommon, and is readily accepted by data managers, manual updating of several page states can present a large burden to the staff and may result in a delay in having the information available or even a serious backup in the workflow.

The ability of a computer system to update a page's state automatically based on the data requires that the system know exactly which page the data came from. There are some data management computer systems that are heavily page based and closely link and store the data as a "page" throughout the data management process. In other systems, the data is stored independent of the page layout (though related, of course) to aid in standardization and pooling of data across studies. In those systems, the link to the paper page may need to be stored with the data (e.g., by entering the page number along with patient identifying information) or through the use of a unique document ID stored with the data.

The latter case is just a simplification of the first: the unique document ID is associated with patient identifying information and a specific page number when the page is first received. This document ID alone is then used to link data to the original page. Because of its simplicity, this method is used even when the page header information is also stored with the data. Note that the document ID is usually a number or barcode and that it could have information such as page and protocol number encoded in it, but a simple sequential number associated with page information on receipt works just as well and provides flexibility.

Tracking challenges

Tracking systems and their associated processes need to be able to manage a set of typical situations that arise with CRFs:

- Repeating pages with the same page number
- Pages with no data
- Duplicate pages
- Pages with no page number

Repeating pages

Repeating pages are those in which there is more than one copy of a page with the same page number. Repeating pages occur most frequently with pages such as concomitant medications or adverse event (AE) pages where the sponsor may not know how many copies are required to capture all the information obtained from the patient and so provides each site with several identical copies. Other common examples of repeating pages are those that capture hospitalization information or drug dosing.

Sometimes the CRF designer will guess an upper limit and repeat those pages — each its own page number (e.g., pages 140, 141, and 142 may all be AE pages). A more common design is to give these pages a single, base page number and provide a blank "repeat" or "sequence" field for the page. The site fills in the blank with a number or letter such as:

140.0, 140.1, 140.2

or

140, 140a, 140b

The database design associated with these fields often divides the page number into two fields: one that is the page and another that is a sequence number, as in page=14, sequence=2. Whether it is one field or two, the tracking system would have to handle a base page 140 with multiple occurrences of that page for a single patient.

Pages with no data

Some pages in a CRF booklet will not have data to enter into the database. Some, such as pages designed to hold copies of specimen labels, are designed to have no data but the sponsor does expect to receive them as part of the study. In other cases, a patient may miss an entire visit or the study design may call for alternate pages to be used in special circumstances. In those examples, the site is frequently instructed to send in the empty pages or not-applicable pages with a line drawn through them and "not done" or "no data" written on them. If data is being tracked through entry, repeated double-checking of why data from those pages is missing can be avoided by marking these pages as "no data" pages when they are received or when they arrive at first entry.

Duplicate pages

No matter how well designed the CRF is or how carefully monitors instruct the sites, sites seem to find ways to send in duplicate pages for a patient. Some actual examples help illustrate what can happen:

- The site notices they filled out a form incorrectly, but it was already collected. So, they fill out a new one transcribing much of the data but correcting some of the data.
- The site sends in a page marked as having "no data," realizes they made a mistake, but now the page has a line through it, so they fill out a new one. The monitor collects both.

Ideally, the tracking system will identify duplicate (nonrepeating) pages when they are logged in. When problems are caught early in the process, they are usually much easier to fix. Unfortunately, not all tracking systems catch duplicates early and so it falls to data management and/or statistical reports to identify the problem further down the road. Once duplicate pages are identified, it is usually necessary to remove one of them from the system.

Studies without page numbers

Historically, not all studies had page numbers on all the CRF pages. Some of these studies did not follow the typical structure where visits happen in a predefined sequence ending with a termination page. Studies with repeated applications of a treatment or dosing (possibly by the patient at home) are one example. In other cases, the CRF pages were not numbered to reduce the number of unique page templates needed for printing — that used to reduce the cost significantly. In some of those studies, a page template name identified the kind of page (e.g., "Demog" page, "PE" page, "Lab" page, and so forth) and the pages repeated in visits or cycles. In others, the unique document identifier was deemed sufficient to identify and track the page.

With advances in printing and because of the convenience of page numbers, we see this much less frequently. In fact, most tracking systems require a page number. Should a CRF design arise without the normal page numbers, consider carefully how (if at all), it could be tracked with existing tracking methods.

Missing pages reports

There are two kinds of missing pages reports and they have separate goals. Data management groups have long used the first kind of report in which a list of pages is checked against the clinical database to ensure that all pages that have been received have been entered into the database. These reports only make sense if there is a list somewhere (paper or electronic) of pages that have been received by the group. When tracking is only done at the time of first entry, a reconciliation of pages received to pages entered is not possible and other procedures must be in place to ensure that no data was inadvertently overlooked.

The second kind of missing pages report lists pages that are expected but "missing" by patient. This information is used by CRAs and monitors to determine whether there are pages at a site that should be collected at an upcoming visit or pages that were missed during a previous visit. For companies that use paper CRFs, data management is usually responsible for providing this information to the clinical group. Ideally, the programmers creating these reports will use existing tracking and database objects and data so that data management need not duplicate information into yet another table and also so that the program need not be customized for every study. In any case, the program will only be able to report missing pages if the list of expected pages is clearly defined.

What pages do you expect?

When setting up a missing pages report, nearly every group starts with a list of all the pages of the CRF for each patient for the entire study and tags them as "expected." Site monitors and CRAs stop using these reports almost immediately because they are over-reporting. In reality, we don't expect all the pages for a given patient at once, we only expect pages up to the patient's most recent visit. One simple modification can make a big improvement here: the program can expect pages only through the patient's highest visit logged into tracking. That is, if there are any pages logged in for a patient in visit 2, then the report expects all required pages through visit 2 but does not expect visit 3. This way, the monitor will easily notice if the physical exam page from the first visit was missing. Taking this another step, the program could be configured to expect visit 3 two weeks after the visit 2 date (plus a buffer to permit monitoring).

Another problem in over-reporting occurs when a patient terminates from the study early. In this case, the report should only list required pages up through the last visit plus any termination pages. Pages from visits beyond the termination visit are not typically collected and should not be considered "missing." If there is a way to identify a termination page or pages in the list of expected pages, the reporting program can look for that page and apply the appropriate logic for considering a page to be missing.

Alternate visits pose a huge problem to missing page reports. Some study designs have the patient follow an alternate visit if certain conditions are met. For example, consider the case of a protocol that says: if certain test results come up positive, the patient follows "Alternate Visit 1" rather than the normal "Day 15" and then goes to "Alternate Visit Follow-up" instead of "Day 30" after which the patient resumes the normal schedule. In this case, to avoid writing custom missing pages reports for this study, consider having the program require all pages for an alternate visit if one of the pages in that visit shows up. Also instruct the site to send in the "Day 15" pages with a line through and marked as "not applicable" or "no data." Even though this is a bit extra work for the site and monitor, the missing pages report will run appropriately because the required "Day 15" pages are there and all of the alternate pages are accounted for. With a little care, no visit or page will be inadvertently overlooked. That assurance justifies the extra work!

Reporting on missing pages

The more advanced, and useful, versions of missing pages reports described above require visit information. This implies that the tracking system either tracks the visit information explicitly or the program brings it in from other sources. It is also worth pointing out that just listing page numbers on these reports is not as helpful as including a brief text describing what kind of page it is. The information that patient 1001001 is missing page 23, the "Vital Signs" from Visit 2, is more helpful to the site monitor than just reporting that patient 1001001 is missing page 23.

Tracking query forms

Discrepancies are any problems with the data that need to be resolved. Some of these are sent to investigator sites on a special form often called a query form (see Chapter 7). Because the investigator will correct and provide data on the query form, it must be tracked to ensure that no correction is lost. Query forms are records of patient data just as the CRFs are. In some cases the discrepancy management system will track the query forms as part of discrepancy management and processing; in other systems, the same tracking system used for CRFs can track the forms.

The goals for tracking query forms are the same as those for CRFs: to ensure that no data is lost and to provide information on the status of the data in the system. This tracking information regarding query forms and the associated data is critical to a study. A study cannot be locked for analysis until all open discrepancies and queries are accounted for, if not resolved. Although the goals for tracking query forms are the same as those for tracking CRFs, the different workflow for query forms introduces complications. Some possible workflow differences include:

- A query form is often explicitly tracked as "sent to the site," independent of when it was generated.
- Query forms may have no changes to data on them, so they may be filed immediately. (That is, the data is "okay as is.")
- There is no second entry pass when data changes are present but there may be visual verification.

To further complicate the flow and tracking, some data management groups use a query form that lists multiple discrepancies, which can refer to several CRF pages for that patient. The difference between workflow for CRFs and query forms and the actual contents of the query form will determine whether or not the CRF tracking system can handle both or if two systems are needed.

CROs and tracking

CROs frequently have better tracking systems than sponsor firms because they need them. CROs not only need to track the CRFs with extreme care to avoid loss, but they also need detailed metrics on the data management process for billing and future proposals. On the other hand, the CRO data management groups may not understand the expected page requirements as well as the sponsor and they may miss pages that are required. Having the sponsor data management or clinical group check missing page reports from the CRO can help identify this issue early in the study.

There are also cases where the CRO will either receive CRFs from the sponsor or where the CRO will receive the CRFs from sites but send them during the course of the study to the sponsor. Either of these cases calls for tracking on both sides. Periodic reconciliation will help ensure that no CRFs or query forms were lost in transit.

Quality assurance and quality control

Tracking of CRFs and query forms is a critical component of a quality system for data management as it ensures integrity and accuracy of the data. As with all quality systems, documentation is critical. Usually an electronic database with appropriate reports is sufficient to indicate tracking is taking place. However, it may be necessary to show some documentation (paper or electronic) that data management staff is actually using the tracking reports to ensure that all data is processed. Discrepancies issued when pages or data is missing are one example of such documentation. Printed and signed reports generated at the close of the study are another.

Tracking also can be used to assist in the quality control audits of CRF data against database values (see Chapter 5). A good tracking system can easily produce lists of pages using various criteria such as:

- Random selection across all pages totaling 10%
- Selection of 10% from each investigator site
- All AE pages
- All pages 14, 21, and 35

The lists of pages may be used to call up images using a document ID or they may include investigator and patient numbers for quick retrieval from a paper filing system. A company might even opt to update a tracking system field for those pages that were included in an audit of data.

SOPs for tracking

An SOP should be in place to require CRF tracking. The actual procedure to follow may be outlined in a separate tracking SOP or referenced in some other SOP or guideline such as that governing CRF workflow. Because of variations in the way tracking systems can be used, data management groups should consider a detailed guideline that outlines what workflow states are to be captured and what kinds of documentation is required to demonstrate appropriate use of tracking. The SOP or guideline can also explain company policy on the special tracking problems described above. The information can also be recorded in the data management plan.

Tracking throughout the process

Tracking, unfortunately, is often an add-on application to data management systems, which is a shame, since a good tracking system can support and make more efficient the entire data management process. A close integration to data management systems makes more automatic updates of page states possible and supports data cleaning efforts. Further integration with discrepancy management systems can tie the whole process together by providing data managers easy access to and information on pages, data, and discrepancies interchangeably.

chapter seven

Cleaning data

The biggest job for any data management group running a paper based trial is not the entry of the data into a clinical database — it is checking the data for discrepancies and getting the data cleaned up. Discrepancies are *any* inconsistencies in the clinical data that require research. Discrepancies may be identified manually at any point during processing when someone reviews either the case report form (CRF) or the data. Most commonly, they are identified by the data management system automatically at entry or after entry via rules defining acceptable data. Discrepancies may also be identified through reporting or analysis in systems external to the data management application.

Each discrepancy is registered or stored in some way until it can be resolved. The process or system to store discrepancies can be called a discrepancy management system. Originally, and perhaps for small studies still, this was done using paper listings and copies of queries sent to sites for resolution. This manual tracking quickly becomes unwieldy. Today, all commercial clinical data management (CDM) systems support the identification and tracking of discrepancies. The discrepancy management portion of CDM systems stores the discrepancy, tracks its status, and records its resolution or type of resolution.

A discrepancy can often be resolved by internal groups, such as the data management group or clinical research associates (CRAs), but at least some portion will need to be resolved by the investigator. Discrepancies that are sent to the sites for resolution are often called "queries." Most commonly, companies send these queries to sites on special query forms that require tracking, just as CRFs do (see Chapter 6). Newer systems may notify investigators of queries via e-mail or special faxes. In electronic data capture systems, queries appear in the same system as is used to collect the data. When forms are used, the site resolves the query by writing directly on the query form and returning that form to the data management group.

Data management updates the discrepancy management system with the kind of resolution for each discrepancy or query. When resolution of a discrepancy takes the form of a corrected value, data management must also

61

update the stored data. Some discrepancy management systems can correct the value in the database at the same time the query is resolved; others require a separate edit to the database.

In this chapter, we detail each of the main aspects of discrepancy management: identifying discrepancies, managing queries, and resolving both queries and discrepancies.

Identifying discrepancies

Discrepancies come from several sources:

- Manual review of data and CRFs by clinical or data management
- Computerized checks of data by the data management system or entry application
- Computerized checks or analysis by data management or biostatistics using external systems

These checks to identify discrepancies are frequently called "edit checks." In order to perform the same checks on all the data consistently throughout the course of the study, data management groups create a list of checks at the start of the study, often called an "edit check specification." (The term "data validation procedures" is also common.) These specifications typically take the form of tables or Excel spreadsheets with one row per check. Each check is identified by the CRF page and/or the module or table in which the value being checked appears. The logic of the check is given in a way understandable to all readers (i.e., in English, not programming language). There is also a message that will be appear when the check finds a discrepancy and there is usually an indicator if this is an automatic check, manual review, external check, or any other checking methods that may be used. See Figure 7.1 for an example of an edit check specification table.

The kinds of checks found in an edit check specification can be categorized as follows:

- Missing values (e.g., dose is missing)
- Simple range checks (e.g., dose must be between 100 and 500 mg)
- Logical inconsistencies (e.g., "no hospitalizations" is checked but a date of hospitalization is given)
- Checks across modules (e.g., adverse event (AE) action taken says "study termination" but the study termination pages does not list AE as a cause of termination)
- Protocol violations (e.g., time when blood sample is drawn is after study drug taken and should be before, per protocol)

A few companies have also developed algorithms that look for fraud, but this is still quite rare. (Figure 7.2 lists these typical checks, but grouped into

Page Number	Module	Check Name	Edit Check	Edit Check Message	Method
1	**DEMOG**	DOBD_MISSING	Date of birth is missing or incomplete.	The subject's date of birth is missing or is incomplete. Please clarify.	Auto
		AGE_RANGE	Subject is less than 18 years old.	Based upon the date of birth 'dob date', the subject is less than 18 years old. Please verify date of birth.	Auto
		SEX_MISSING	Sex is missing or more than one box is marked.	Sex is missing or more than one box is marked. Please clarify.	Auto
		ETHNIC_MISSING	Ethnicity is missing or more than one box is marked.	Ethnicity is missing or more than one box is marked. Please clarify.	Auto
		ETHNIC_1	Ethnicity is 'Other', but a specification is missing.	Ethnicity is marked "Other", however, the other ethnicity is not specified. Please specify the ethnicity.	Auto
		ETHNIC_2	Ethnicity is not 'Other', but a specification is provided (when none of boxes is marked).	Ethnicity is not marked "Other", however, an ethnicity is specified. Please clarify.	Auto

Figure 7.1 Example of an edit check specification table for some demographics information.

different categories.) For a medium-sized CRF and a study of medium complexity, 400 separate checks would not be unusual and it could well be significantly more.

Manual review

At some firms, data managers go over the CRF before it is sent to data entry but the value of this initial review is questionable (this is discussed further in Chapter 5). Data entry staff can be trained to identify significant problems that would prevent entry of an entire page (such as a missing patient ID, which is a far more common occurrence than one would think). Handwriting that is hard to read is more properly sent through the entry process where it will be flagged if it cannot be deciphered by entry staff rather than having a single data manager decide what the value *should* be. In general, letting discrepancies be identified by the appropriate source leads to better quality and allows valuable senior data managers to focus on the actual problems found, rather than requiring them to look at all the pages hunting for possible problems.

A kind of manual review that *does* bring a great deal of value is the kind that takes place not just after entry of a single patient's data but after a significant amount of data across patients has been entered. This is often called a listing review. Listings of text fields are a very common kind of listing review. Data managers use these listings to identify unusual texts that have passed entry but do not appear to make sense. Often the entry staff is focused on responses number by number or letter by letter and so they miss obvious phrases. Data managers can step back and look at a whole phrase. One actual example is that two entry operators entered the phrase "Injured tue" because both of them saw a "u" in the second word. The data manager reviewing text listings found this phrase odd and by reviewing the original CRF was able to make the appropriate change to "Injured toe."

Clinical team members (e.g., CRAs) are also asked to review texts looking for medical problems or inconsistencies because that kind of review would be inappropriate for data managers without a medical background to perform. They also look for monitoring problems such as medications listed in medical history rather than in the concomitant medications list. They may cross check medications against AEs, and so forth.

Data managers and statisticians may manually review certain key numeric values and dates looking for odd patterns or inconsistencies that have not been programmed into the edit checks. Statisticians may also run some simple analyses looking for outliers. There is no value in having anyone manually recheck data in the same way as a programmed edit check unless there is suspicion that the program is running incorrectly.

Whatever the source of the manual discrepancy, it must be registered in the system so it can be tracked. In order to enforce careful checking and consistency, companies typically have data managers create the actual discrepancies regardless of who identifies them. The data management group

Completeness and consistency:

- Checks for empty fields
- Cooking for all related items
- Cross-checking values

Real-world checks:

- Range checks
- Discrete value checks
- One value greater/less than/equal to another

Quality control:

- Are dates in a logical sequence?
- Is header information consistent?
- Any missing visits or pages?

Compliance:

- Are visits in compliance with protocol?
- Inclusion/exclusion criteria met?
- Procedures performed in the proper order?

Safety:

- Checking laboratory values against normals
- Comparison of values over time

Others:
- Fraud

Figure 7.2. Typical kinds of checks used to identify discrepancies in clinical data.

must be very careful to review all existing discrepancies associated with the same data before creating a manual discrepancy and sending it to the site as a query. Sites find it very annoying when they get two queries that ask them the same thing, as might happen if two different people saw the same problem during different kinds of review.

Entry problems

Data managers tend not to put many field or page-level checks in entry applications or entry screens if double entry is being used (see Chapter 5). If there are checks, these are set up so that entry staff receives a warning but can continue to enter and store the value data anyway. Entry staff should usually be able to enter a value on the CRF as it is and problems should be identified by the edit check programs post entry. If they cannot enter the value, some groups have the entry operator leave the field blank because a missing value check will flag it. Sometimes, companies use sticky notes and one wonders what happens when they happen to come off! Some entry systems allow the entry operator to electronically flag the data for additional review. Given the possible variations for dealing with data that cannot be entered, clear processes must be in place in every data management group to ensure that data is later reviewed.

Automatic checks

Despite the attention we have just given to manual checks, only a small percentage of the checks listed in an edit specification will be manual. Most types of edit checks can be programmed and are more reliable if they are automatic. Perhaps 80% of the automatic checks for a given protocol will fall into the missing values, simple range check, and inconsistency detection categories. Depending on the data management system, these can often be defined (programmed) by experienced data managers. The remaining checks would be considered more complex and if they cross patients, datasets, or pages, a programmer experienced with the underlying database may need to define them.

External system checks

Systems external to the data management application are frequently used to review and analyze clinical data. The data management system may not be able to support checks across patient records, visits, and pages (and even if it does, CDM staff may not have expertise to write those checks), so other packages such as SAS® are used. These applications may be run by data management specifically to check data, or they may be used by other groups to review data and begin analysis.

Problem data may become apparent from any of these reports, analyses, or graphs and must also be registered as a discrepancy. Just as with the discrepancies that arise during listing reviews, data managers usually register these discrepancies manually. It is worth noting, however, that there are systems where discrepancies identified externally can be formatted and automatically loaded into the discrepancy management portion of the CDM system.

Managing discrepancies

All discrepancies that are identified automatically by the system are reviewed by a data manager familiar with the edit check specifications and also with the CRF. It is common for a large percentage of discrepancies to be resolved internally. For a study of medium complexity with several or many sites, we can very roughly estimate one discrepancy per CRF page. Of those, from 60% to 70% will be resolved internally by inspection of the CRF and related data. The remaining ones will be sent to the investigator sites as queries for resolution.

Resolving discrepancies internally

It may come as a surprise to someone unfamiliar with the process that many discrepancies can be resolved internally. These are resolved by experienced data managers through inspection of the CRF. A common example of a problem that might generate many discrepancies that are resolved internally is found in questionnaire data. Data managers will typically require that each response in the questionnaire be "not-missing." However, patients do skip questions and leave them blank or mark two boxes. Questionnaire data is often not queried because the response must reflect the patient's feelings on the day the answer is given. A data manager will review a discrepancy raised by missing questionnaire data and confirm that it really is blank on the CRF and was not inadvertently left blank during the entry process. The data manager then closes the discrepancy with an "ok as is" final status of resolution.

Another example of resolving discrepancies internally comes from barely legible values. Data entry staff may have flagged a field as illegible, or first- and second-pass entries may have been different. A data manager who reviews the CRF in the context of that and other pages may be able to read the value without guessing. (That is critical, of course: guessing is not allowed.) When in doubt, a discrepancy should always be sent to the site asking for clarification of the value.

Nearly all data management groups allow data managers to correct certain inconsistencies in the data. These are often called self evident corrections (SECs). The kinds of changes permitted are tightly restricted and limited to a study specific, predefined list. The changes a data manager is allowed to make would not usually involve any changes to actual data or result values. Data that provide context and whose correct value can be unequivocally determined may be changed. Typical examples of SECs include:

- Medications are listed on the page but the box saying "Are there any medications" is blank; data managers can mark the box as "yes." The reverse is not permitted! Many other indicator boxes of this kind lend themselves to allowing a self evident correction.
- If the patient ID is blank or incorrect but the page was sent in context with other data from that patient and other values such as initials are consistent, then the patient ID can be corrected.
- Dates occurring in January are sometimes accidentally given the preceding year. When there is no question as to the correct year value, data managers may change it.

While nearly all data management groups allow such self evident corrections — and the percentage of discrepancies that these corrections address is significant — companies are not in agreement on how to handle the regulation ICH GCP section 8.3.15 that requires the site be aware of "… all changes/additions or corrections made to CRF after initial data were recorded." Some data management groups send the list of SECs to the investigators at the start of the study informing them of the changes that *will be* made. Other groups send a specific list of changes at the end of the study to each investigator showing changes that *were* made. A few companies do both. These approaches all seem to satisfy the requirements, but feelings one way or the other about what is "correct" run very strong. (It should be noted that in recent informal surveys at data management meetings, the majority of companies seem to be leaning toward the notification at the start of the study.)

It is very important to understand that these data management SECs are specifically *not* data entry guidelines. If the changes were implemented as data entry guidelines and were made at the time of first entry, they would not have an audit trail. By allowing the data to raise a discrepancy, the change in the data is clearly identified with a reason for change, has a person associated with the actual edit, and is usually reviewed by a second person.

Anything that cannot be resolved by data management is a candidate for being sent to the site as a query. At some companies, CRAs also review these candidate queries. While they are never permitted to make changes to data, they are sometimes permitted to mark a query as "Confirmed as is" if they have prior documentation of that value in the form of a copy of a source document or as a specific reference in a visit report. For example, a CRA may have noted an unusual lab value during a monitoring visit and researched it. If that research is documented, the CRA may be permitted to return the query to data management without getting further site input. It must be noted that not all regulatory groups permit this kind of discrepancy resolution but CRAs, data management, and the sites all like it because it avoids at least some unnecessary queries.

Turning a discrepancy into a query

Once new discrepancies have been thoroughly reviewed, those that have not been resolved internally will require site resolution. These will be sent to the appropriate site, usually on a special form we will call a query form. (Other common names for this form are "Discrepancy Clarification Form" or "Data Correction Form.") These forms have many different names but the same purpose: they present the discrepancy in a way understandable to the site and likely to lead to clear resolution.

When the edit checks were specified, they had error texts associated with them. Ideally, these texts would have been carefully crafted to avoid references to database terms or confusing logic. This way they would be automatically and consistently assigned to the same kinds of discrepancies. Realistically, data managers often tailor the message for some portion of the discrepancies before they are sent in order to make them clear and specific to the case in question. While some of this should be encouraged, it should not be necessary to tailor all automatic discrepancy texts.

Also, while editing these messages, data managers should be carefully instructed to avoid leading questions. For example, in the case of an illegible value, the data manager should not write: "Was the value meant to be 23?" Instead, the message should say the value was not legible and could the site please provide the correct value. This way, the site must go to the source document and check the value rather than just automatically say "yes." Other cases of leading questions are less clear and are sometimes permitted. In the case of dates, for example, some companies will permit a discrepancy message to read something like: "Confirm that the year is 2005." Data managers must have clear guidelines around messages to avoid inadvertently violating company policy on leading questions!

In most data management systems today, the query forms are created automatically when the discrepancy is ready to send. The discrepancies will always belong to a single site and nearly always a single patient, but they may have:

- Multiple queries over multiple CRF pages
- Multiple queries referring to a single CRF page only
- A single query only

Entering only discrepancies for a single patient and page combination on a query form greatly increases the number of forms sent to the site but it does simplify tracking, filing, and imaging. (For example, forms with discrepancies for a single page only can be electronically "stapled" to a CRF image for easy review.)

Different firms, and sometimes different groups within a single firm, may prefer a different organization of queries. They are often influenced by specific investigators who strongly favor one approach over another and they may be limited in what they can choose by their data management system.

Resolving queries

The query form, once produced, is delivered to the site via fax, paper mail, the CRA in person, or e-mail. The site researches the discrepancies and provides resolutions using the company-specified method. For paper based processes, the site typically writes the resolution into a spot on the query form, signs and dates it, and files it with the patient binders at the site. (Responses on query forms must be treated by both the site and the sponsor just as CRFs are because they contain original site data.)

Getting signatures

"Sign and date" does not sound controversial, but it is. Some companies require that the principal investigator (PI) sign each discrepancy. In this case, a subinvestigator is permitted to sign only if that investigator has been assigned this responsibility in the site's regulatory paperwork. Nearly every company that requires PI signature runs into the problem of investigators being away for a long time on vacation or business so that they cannot sign query forms. This problem is particularly serious as a study lock approaches. Despite the practical problems for data management and the CRAs who work with the sites, many regulatory groups insist that this procedure is the *only* way that the sponsor can be sure the principal investigator is personally aware of all data changes as per ICH GCP section 8 (see earlier discussion in this chapter).

Some other companies take a different approach and allow a study coordinator to take responsibility for, and sign, some or all of the resolutions on query forms. These companies then meet the requirement to make sure the PI is aware of all CRF changes by sending the changes at the end of the study or as the patient closes out. The changes may be in the form of lists of changed values or as copies of updated CRFs ("working copies") that show the changes. The PI is asked to sign a form saying that he is aware of all the data. This procedure does generally allow for faster turnaround on getting discrepancy resolutions but brings up the question of whether the investigator does, in truth, review the changes before signing off.

Applying the resolution

When a site provides the resolution to a discrepancy on a query form, they may write a paragraph explaining the correct action or justifying a value, and a CRA or data manager may need to interpret the response to determine what action to take. It may even be necessary to resend the query to get clarification on the resolution! Because of problems in interpreting site responses, and because site responses may hint at a medical issue or even contain a subtle protocol violation, many companies have CRAs review all queries as they come in from the sites. This is not a universal approach but anecdotal information indicates that it produces positive results in quality of the data and improves safety surveillance for the companies that try it.

For those queries that require a change to data or provide a missing value, the value is usually applied via an edit feature using normal data entry screens. As noted in Chapter 5, correction or editing of clinical data to reflect a resolution generally follows a different path from that of initial entry of the data. In particular, data management systems often don't support second entry of edits, so many companies require a visual review of the edits or a comparison of the audit trail of the database against the query form to confirm that the change was made correctly. Some data management systems support a process whereby the data manager supplies a correct value for a field as a proposed action at the time the resolution type (or status) is recorded for the discrepancy. This proposed action may be reviewed before it is actually applied. The review of the edit or review of the proposed action reflects the fact that many companies were finding that errors were being introduced more through the edit process than through the initial entry process, clearly indicating that extra attention is needed to ensure accuracy in these steps.

After edits are made, it is essential to rerun all cleaning rules over the data as it is very common for updates to the data, as part of a discrepancy resolution, to cause some other discrepancy to be raised!

The site response to a query may not result in a change to the data. The original value may really be as reported on the CRF or it may not be possible to obtain a response or value. These responses must still be logged into the discrepancy management system so that the discrepancy is closed. Most discrepancy systems will check for duplicates so that even though the patient's data would still raise a discrepancy, the system recognizes that it has already been raised (and closed) and will not raise it again.

Quality assurance and quality control

Good discrepancy management systems and processes become involved in both quality assurance and quality control processes. Knowing which changes were made and why they were made is an integral part of quality assurance (QA) practices and is required by regulations. While data management systems must have an audit trail that includes a reason for each change, the discrepancy management system provides more detail on the steps taken to resolve each issue.

Feedback is another element of QA. When discrepancies and resolutions are reviewed, the information can be fed back to the source. This can, for example, improve collection of data during the study when site training is improved and can lead to improvements in data capture and collection methods in future studies.

Quality control of entered data usually takes the form of data audits against the CRF. Discrepancy management information and associated query forms should be able to account for differences between the data in the database and the original CRF. As part of normal audits or as a separate task, resolutions that lead to database edits should be audited. Separately, a review of the data management system audit trail against the discrepancy-system records should show that no changes were made to clinical data without a link to a known discrepancy.

Being able to differentiate between different kinds of resolutions can provide helpful metrics. Discrepancy management and query resolution is a large and resource-intensive part of data management for paper trails. Knowing the expected number of discrepancies, the percentage that will be closed by data management, and the percentage requiring a site query will be critical to staffing and budgeting for large studies. Figure 7.3 shows some examples of discrepancy states, resolution types, and resolution sources. While the discrepancy management system may impose limitations on possible values, choosing options that permit counting the different ways of resolving a discrepancy is essential to providing those metrics.

Open discrepancy states:
- Identified or registered (new)
- Reviewed and still open
- Sent to site
- Duplicate or linked
- Received from the site (but not yet reviewed)

Resolution types:
- Resolved (with data from site)
- As is (i.e., not a problem)
- Cannot be resolved (but incorrect)
- Data management SEC

Resolution sources:
- CRA
- Data management
- Site, by phone
- Site, by query form

Figure 7.3 Some examples of discrepancy states, resolution types, and sources of a resolution that may be used by discrepancy management systems.

SOPs for discrepancy management

SOPs for discrepancy management vary in their level of detail. Some are written at a very high level that is not dependent on the individual software system and only provides general guidelines about who can make corrections and how the corrections are to be received and recorded. Other procedures in the form of guidelines or manuals may provide details as to the process of identifying and resolving discrepancies that is system- or application-dependent and include a discussion on how to customize messages and link related discrepancies and properly identify the final resolution.

Many data management groups also have study specific discrepancy-management guidelines that help clarify special handling beyond what is in the edit specifications. This sort of document is a good place to record what site notations or other documentation will be accepted to close a discrepancy. For example, if a CRF module does not have a not-done box because a value is always expected, but the study turns out otherwise and sites are writing in "Not Done," then it may be permissible to close the discrepancy for missing values in the module with an "ok as is" or "not available" sort of resolution. The study specific document can also describe handling for different CRF page versions and so on. In short, anything that is not clear from the edit specifications or any special handling that develops as the study progresses can be well documented in study specific discrepancy management guidelines or directly in the data management plan.

Making a difference

Several studies have shown that identifying discrepancies early on and continuously throughout the process of data management leads to better-quality data and faster closure of studies. When discrepancies are identified early in the study, it is often possible to uncover problems with a field on the CRF or misunderstandings at a particular site. Clarifications or further training that addresses those problems can prevent the same discrepancies from occurring throughout the entire study. This expectation of running edit checks soon after the first patient data begin to arrive is an industry standard.

Another way to make a difference is to take time at the end of a study to review discrepancy metrics:

- What kind of checks on what kinds of fields failed most frequently
- What percentage of discrepancies are resolved in house
- What percentage of queries to sites require data changes
- What queries take the longest to resolve

These numbers can improve the next CRF, the next edit check specification, the next set of SECs, and the next site training. Do not just count the numbers; do something with them.

Discrepancy management and query resolution is such a large part of the data management process in bigger trials that even small improvements in process and systems can have a huge impact on reducing needed resources and shortening timelines. It is worth reviewing the process in detail every few years to make sure that procedures still make sense and make efficient use of the computer applications being used.

chapter eight

Managing laboratory data

Laboratory data is the name given to the class of data that includes blood chemistry, hematology, lipids, and urinalysis values (see Figure 8.1). Lab data for any given study may also include cultures, microbiology, virology, and assays specific to the protocol. Studies collect lab data to provide information on the efficacy and safety of the medication and may also use it in the screening of patients. Nearly all studies have at least some lab data. Sometimes the values are written on the case report form (CRF). In other cases, the values are obtained from a central laboratory that supplies the results in the form of an electronic file.

Whatever the source, managing the lab data and all the associated values frequently represent a good sized portion of the data management effort for a study. Some of this is due to the sheer volume of the result data, and the rest is due to the numerous tasks that are associated with managing this data. Many data management groups designate one or more staff members as lab data administrators or coordinators. When viewing all of the tasks that need to be managed with lab data, it is easy to see why someone may take this on as a full-time assignment. Lab data administrators:

- Provide input into CRF and eCRF design
- Answer study setup questions
- Coordinate with central laboratories
- Specify or even write loading programs (for electronic files)
- Check file formats and track data deliveries (for electronic files)
- Oversee entry questions (for CRF data)
- Resolve questions of units
- Run and/or review cleaning checks
- Check for patterns in the data
- Resolve discrepancies
- Keep normal range data current

In this chapter, we will look at some of the key areas that lab data administrators need to understand. We will first look at how lab data and the

75

Blood Chemistry	Hematology	Urinalysis
GLUCOSE	WBC	pH
CREATININE	HEMOGLOBIN	GLUCOSE
SGOT	HEMATACRIT	KETONES
SGPT	BASOPHILS	ALBUMIN
BILIRUBIN	PLATELETS	WBC

Figure 8.1 Examples of values generally called lab data. Note that some assays, such as WBC, show up in more than one group. Be aware that these are *not* the same values. They measure different things and have different units.

associated units are stored and how that data is checked and cleaned. Then, because lab data is often provided by central labs in electronic files, we will discuss central labs and the loading of those electronic files.

Storing lab data

When they set up database structures for a study, database designers also prepare the structures to store lab data and associated information. As we saw in Chapter 3, database tables may be structured in a tall-skinny (normalized) or short-fat format. In the tall-skinny format, there are fewer columns, and data is collected in many rows. In the short-fat format, there is one column for each piece of data collected. Lab data lends itself particularly well to a tall-skinny format, despite the fact that it makes some kinds of queries and checks more complex.

Advantages of the tall-skinny format

The reasons most companies prefer the tall-skinny format for lab data include:

- The need to store information in addition to the actual test result
- Ease of checking against normal ranges
- The structure allows for flexibility in reporting and analysis
- Loading routines for electronic files are simpler

All these points are worth exploring in further detail.

The need to store information in addition to the test result is probably the overwhelming reason to use a tall-skinny format. One common CRF page design for collecting lab data has a single field next to the name of each lab test where someone from the site writes in the result and next to that might be a box to indicate if the site finds this value to be clinically abnormal. There may even be a text field associated with "if abnormal." Besides the results and the "abnormal" indicators, lab results have further additional data associated with them, some of which are printed on the page and some of which are calculated or derived. Units are often preprinted on the page, yet they should always be stored with the data in the database (see later). Derived or calculated data may include test values converted to standard units. If a tall-skinny format is used to store the result fields for abnormal, and then also units and a standardized result, this structure (a table or record) would have six columns; a short-fat format would have the number of columns equal to five times the number of tests. Figure 8.2 shows a tall-skinny lab table and a short-fat lab table for the case of the four fields only per lab test only.

Normal ranges for laboratory values are nearly always stored in the tall-skinny format when they are collected (see later). Checking routines that compare the test results against the normal range for that test are easiest to create when the two structures are in the same format. If both are in the tall-skinny format, checking programs can be based on simple database joins.

The characteristics of relational databases and some analysis packages mean that the tall-skinny format provides an extra level of flexibility in creating reports. The tall-skinny format can be easily "denormalized" to present the data in a short-fat format. However, taking a short-fat format and converting it to the tall-skinny presentation requires more complex programming.

Tall-skinny format:

Test_name	Test_result	Units	Standard_ result
WBC		10*3	
HEMOGLOBIN		g/dl	
HEMATOCRIT		%	
BASOPHILS		%	
PLATELETS		/mm*3	

Short-fat format:

WBC	WBC_UNIT	STD_WBC	HEMOGLOBIN	HEMOGLOBIN _UNIT	STD_ HEMOGLOBIN

HEMATOCRIT	HEMATOCRIT _UNIT	STD_HEMA- TOCRIT	BASOPHIL	BASOPHIL_ UNIT	STD_BASO- PHIL

PLATELETS	PLATELETS_ UNIT	STD_PLATE- LETS

Figure 8.2 Lab results with additional fields for units and standardized results stored in a tall-skinny format and a short-fat format. Both kinds of tables would also have columns for header- and patient identifying information, which are not shown.

Loading programs for lab data can be greatly simplified when a tall-skinny format is used. As the data is read from the file, the result is always placed in the same field or column of the database. This column, by definition, must accept all kinds of values, which reduces problems with unexpected value types. Similarly, all the fields or columns for values associated with the result have clearly defined columns. The mapping effort is greatly simplified compared to the case in which each test and associated value goes into a different field or column.

Disadvantages of the tall-skinny format

The main disadvantage of using this type of tall-skinny format is that the characteristics of each column must apply to all of the data to be stored in the column. For the results column, this means that the expected characteristics of the data cannot be enforced. For example, it is not possible to put simple range checks on the results column of a tall-skinny lab table because it contains results from all kinds of tests. In fact, since the results for some tests are text (e.g., "+2" for glucose measured in urinalysis), the column must be of text type. These characteristics also dictate that results cannot be coded. That is, test results that otherwise might be coded (such as platelet estimate: 1=adequate/2=inadequate), would have to be stored as simple values such as: "ADQ" And "INADQ."

Another disadvantage of the tall-skinny format is the extra work introduced when writing checking routines, derivations, and queries. Each check must include the name of the test as part of the logic. That is, a range check on "Hemoglobin" in a short-fat format might read:

hemoglobin >= 11.9 and hemoglobin <=17.0

and in a tall-skinny format as:

test_name="HEMOGLOBIN" AND

(test_result>=11.9 and test_result<=17.0).

It may not look like much additional work, but over the many lab tests common to most studies, errors are bound to occur in checking routines, reports, and queries.

Despite these significant disadvantages, the flexibility of the format seems to have led nearly all data management groups to store lab data in the tall-skinny format.

Identifying lab tests

Whether the lab results are stored in the tall-skinny or the short-fat format, the tests must be identified. In the tall-skinny format, the name of the test (or a code for the name) appears as a data value in the "test name" column. In the short-fat format, the name of the test is used to name a column onto itself (refer again to Figure 8.2).

In both cases, care must be taken to recognize the difference between similarly named results collected in different ways. For example, a test named "Glucose" appears in both blood chemistry tests and urinalysis tests, and they are not the same. Similarly, it might be important to differentiate between values taken in fasting and nonfasting states. Naming the tests differently is the method usually used for assays that appear in more than one grouping of tests. The hematology version of WBC may be called HWBC and the urinalysis version may be called UWBC.

Another approach is to store the groupings separately so that blood chemistry values are separate from hematology values, which are separate from urinalysis values. In this case, simply using the name WBC may be adequate to fully identify the value. Storing the grouped values separately can be implemented by using either tall-skinny or short-fat formats.

Identifying the difference between conditions such as fasting and nonfasting for a test is more difficult. Naming would prove unwieldy in particular for those studies that request one or the other or both. One option is to have an indicator field, which is marked "Fasting" or "Nonfasting." This approach is most easily implemented when using the tall-skinny format, as it would allow for one or the other or even both at different points in the study.

Storing units

Laboratory results stored without applicable units lose much of their long-term value. If the results do not have the associated units stored with them, there are difficulties in checking against normal ranges or comparing data across studies. To avoid these problems, database designers should store the units with the test results even if those units are predefined by the study, preprinted on the CRF, or specified by a central laboratory.

Whether or not the units are preset, the database design and data managers must be prepared to handle results reported in different units. If the unexpected units are an exception, they can be treated as such. However, when there are many sites or different laboratories participating in a study, variation in units will be the norm. When variation is expected, some companies choose to store not only the reported result and applicable unit but also a version of the result converted to a standard unit via calculation. This standardized result may be stored in the database as a derived value or appear only in analysis data sets.

Converting results to a standard unit requires that the biostatisticians decide on their preferred units and specify how to convert each possible combination of tests and units to those standards. It also requires that the units collected with the result be stored consistently. That is, grams per deciliter should be stored consistently as "g/dl" or "gm/dl" — not a mixture of both. A units codelist can help enforce company standards, although using such a codelist may mean that the data entry operator enters or selects a value that is not *exactly* what appears on the CRF. (This can be clearly spelled out and documented in data entry instructions.)

Ranges and normal ranges

It is not unusual for companies to perform two kinds of checks on laboratory data — one simple range check on whether the data is plausible and one to evaluate whether the result is clinically significant. In the first case, a query is issued to clarify with the site that the reported value is correct. The second case may warrant attention and action by the medical monitor to ensure that appropriate actions are taken to guard the health of the patient. Clearly, if a trend is found in clinically significant abnormal results, this is an important piece of information about the safety and efficacy of the drug.

The simple range checks used to issue discrepancies are frequently based on either textbook values or experience with the population in a particular study. These are programmed along with the rest of the cleaning rules for the study. To evaluate whether the result of a particular laboratory test is clinically significant, a medical reviewer must know what the values for that test "normally" are. These "normal" values are generally called "normal ranges" or "normals." The normal range for a particular test depends on the method and equipment used to obtain the result and also may depend on other factors such as sex and age. The normal ranges are supplied by the laboratory performing the analysis.

Laboratory IDs

Because normal ranges depend on the method and equipment used, there must be some way of knowing which results, and which normal ranges, come from which locations. Therefore, a laboratory ID of some kind should be associated with the sample (and so each result) and also with each normal range. In some cases, the laboratory will be the same for all patients in a study. More typically, several laboratories process samples for a single study. Because of the importance of knowing which ranges are associated with which values, it is better not to make assumptions but rather to store the laboratory ID for each sample taken from each patient. For example, although an investigator nearly always uses a given lab, there may be an emergency that requires an alternate lab for a set of patients or a period of time.

Normal range storage

Normal ranges may be stored in the same storage area as the clinical trial data or they may be stored centrally and available to multiple studies. Storing the data centrally reduces the work load to enter and manage the values.

However, care must be taken to ensure that checking programs and appropriate staff can access that data. Also, if the study is archived or transferred, the associated normal ranges might need to be extracted for archive or transfer.

As noted previously, normal range data is usually stored using the tall-skinny format. In addition to the high- and low-range values for the result, the normals data must have the laboratory ID and the units used. If ranges are collected more than once per study or if the normal ranges are stored centrally, an effective date must be available in some way. If there is an age or sex dependence, there must also be columns for that. Figure 8.3 shows one example of a group of fields to store normal ranges in a tall-skinny format.

Checking result values

The purpose of normal ranges is to check the laboratory results of the study and identify any that may not be considered normal. Abnormal laboratory results may indicate a safety problem with the study, or they may simply point to a data problem. Laboratory results are checked against the ranges in a variety of ways to look for both safety and data problems.

Rather than handle lab ranges as part of normal discrepancy checking, some companies "flag" the result as being out of range through fields of the database itself or through special reports. The flag is usually an additional database or report field that can have a value such as "H," "L," or "N" for high, low, or normal values. Out-of-range values can be identified through scanning this field manually or through discrepancy checking programs. When results are scanned manually, it may be necessary to manually register a discrepancy to resolve issues where the problem is due to transcription or unit problems.

Both discrepancy checking and reporting on normal range values focus on a single, specific result. They do not detect when values have changed significantly from the baseline for a single patient nor do they identify trends for all or a subset of patients in a study. This kind of cross-visit and cross-patient checking has traditionally been left to the statisticians to

---

LAB_ID — identifies the source of the normal range values
EFFECTIVE_DATE — date the range became effective
TEST_NAME — name of the lab test; must be consistent with that used in storing patient results
TEST_UNITS — units that apply to the range
SEX — if present, the range is sex-dependent
AGE_LO — if present, the low end of the age range to which the normal values apply
AGE_HI — if present, the high end of the age range to which the normal values apply
NORMAL_LO — low end of the normal range
NORMAL_HI – high end of the normal range

Figure 8.3 An example of a group of fields used to store normal range data in a tall-skinny format. Each field creates a column in the table. This example assumes that some of the ranges will be sex- and age-dependent.

perform. However, in the interest of detecting problems early, some data management groups have been given the task of reviewing the laboratory data using special tools and programs before statisticians look at it. While data managers typically do not have the training to make statistical or medical assessments, they can detect patterns that have not been caught by simple range checks.

Using central labs

In multicenter trials, a central laboratory is frequently used to deal with the complex issues of quality control needed at every laboratory. Good Clinical Practice (GCP) guidelines require that all labs have full documentation, data-audit trails, standard procedures, trained staff, archives of samples and data, and routine quality assurance inspections. The sponsor must be assured that the GCP requirements for every lab in the study are met. Shipping samples to a central laboratory for large trails makes this management more reasonable. It also reduces the variations in the normal ranges that would be expected if several labs were used.

Of course, there are factors to consider for the use of local laboratories including:

- Expertise in particular area, perhaps with an unusual assay
- Need for very fast analysis due to medical need or for screening purposes
- Problems with logistics or cost of sample transportation

In a trail with a single or few sites, the local laboratory may well provide a convenient and cost-effective option.

Using specialty labs

Many companies are developing drugs and devices on the cutting edge of science. This often means that the lab tests or assays they need to perform to determine the efficacy of the treatment are also on the cutting edge. When this is the case, the sponsor will sometimes need to turn to specialized laboratories to perform the tests. All too often, these are small labs or even investigator sites that are not set up with good practices, standard operating procedures (SOPs), and systems that are 21 CFR 11 compliant. The sponsor receives a shipment of data at the end of the study and quickly identifies a raft of problems or inconsistencies and is faced with the question, "How reliable and analyzable is this data?" The sponsor must then consider the question of whether the study must be rerun or whether some other approach can be taken to avoid throwing out the results of the trail!

There are two important steps that sponsors can take ahead of time to help assure a level of confidence in the data: auditing the lab and setting up verification procedures.

Auditing the lab

The sponsor is ultimately responsible for data coming from a laboratory. When central labs are used, companies will typically audit the lab or will refer to a recent past audit. For the most part, this is a cursory audit as large central laboratories are audited constantly and are likely to have reasonable practices and be in compliance with regulations. When a small laboratory or investigator site is needed for a study, the sponsor must audit much more carefully and pay particular attention to the computer systems that will be used for collection and storage of the data. There must be assurance that the data is reliable and reflect the actual results.

In a very common scenario, the lab will run a specialized assay on a sample using some equipment it owns. The equipment is likely to be validated and reliable and it will often print a result. These results may be taped into a lab notebook or filed in some other way. Later, someone at the lab transcribes the result into Microsoft Excel or Access. Neither of these packages is a 21 CFR 11 compliant system if used "as is" out of the box and creating a compliant application based on them is a significant undertaking. If the lab does nothing more than enter the data into a file, there is no security against inadvertent or intentional changes, no audit trail, and no checks to assure accurate transcription.

It is important to note that a lab *can* use these packages if they reliably verify 100% of the data and then immediately lock or store the files on read-only media (such as a CD) to prevent changes. While this is a simple approach, it does take a lot of discipline to satisfy the "reliably" part so that changes are not made after the data has been verified. It comes down to how good the procedures are and how likely laboratory staff are to follow those procedures consistently.

The lab ships the data to the sponsor who may run edit checks or other types of analyses over it. The edit checks are likely to identify discrepancies in the data, so a process must be in place with the laboratory that details how corrections are to be made. Normal query forms may be the best approach here unless there are a large number of changes expected. In that case, it may be more efficient to have the lab correct the original file (verified, of course, to detect inadvertent changes while editing) and resend.

Verifying the data

Another approach to assuring the reliability of specialized lab results is to monitor the data in a way similar to the monitoring of CRF data. In this approach, the lab processes samples and records results according to good procedures (one hopes!) and ships the resulting data as an electronic file to the sponsor. The sponsor then loads or stores the data in the clinical data management system (CDM) where it is then under audit trail. A monitor then receives a listing of the data from the CDM system and possibly also a list of discrepancies that have been raised on the data through the normal edit checks.

The monitor takes those listings to the lab and 100% verifies the listed data against source data. As noted above, the source data could well be printouts taped into lab notebooks. If the monitor identifies an error, the correction is made at the sponsor with appropriate documentation and under audit trail. Whether the lab updates its own copy of the data is up to the lab; in this approach, there is no resending of the data. Because this kind of independent verification is much like the monitoring of CRF data, the level of confidence in that data will be similar to that for CRF data.

Loading lab data

Central labs typically, and local labs increasingly, deliver data to the sponsor in the form of an electronic file. The file layout, record format, and contents vary widely. In Europe, the Association of Clinical Data Managers has made an effort to standardize a file format for laboratory data but elsewhere it remains mostly up to each sponsor to specify a format or take what the lab typically provides. The laboratory data delivered electronically is usually most frequently loaded into the central database at the sponsor but sponsors may opt to maintain the data as read-only SAS files.

Writing loading applications

Loading the lab data into a central database is done either through programs written specifically for each study or by configuring an application. As noted previously, whether users write a program or configure an application that affects clinical data, it should be subject to a validation process. Given the importance of lab data, this should be especially true for applications that load lab data across studies.

The validation process starts with a specification. A mapping of the layout of the electronic file to the database storage structures provides the basis of the specification, which also should include details on how to handle specific problems (examples below). The process continues with the program being written according to good practices or the application being configured according to guidelines and manuals. Documented testing and specific user instructions round out the requirements. Satisfying validation needs adds significantly to the development effort for these loading applications. The more consistent the file structures, the less overall effort required.

Electronic file contents

An electronic file of lab data contains study- and patient identifying information and results and often assessments of, or comments about, the results.

There is "hidden" or assumed information in the file also. In addition to knowing where to find the results for each test, the lab administrator or data manager needs to know this hidden information including:

- How tests are identified (the names used)
- How the patient and lab is identified
- The difference (if any) between missing and "not done"
- What indicates a retest

The possibilities these issues present make clear that loading applications frequently need to go beyond simple transfers of data from a position in a file to a field in a database. For example, if the laboratory uses different test names than those the company uses in the central database, remapping of the names may be required before loading. If the patient identifier used by the lab is not in the standard format of the sponsor, the loading program may have to support an algorithm to construct the sponsor's identifier. If a test is missing or not done, will it be included anyway, or must the loading program check for and create an empty entry? If a retest is performed, is that clear or will the loading program have to check for and handle duplicate tests?

When receiving data files, it is critically important to know if the file contains only the data recorded since the last delivery or all of the data recorded to that point. The incremental method is usually easier to manage but does entail the checking for duplicate tests. Complete transfers can simplify matters if the existing data can be completely replaced. Unfortunately, when data is replaced at each transfer, keeping connections to discrepancies raised on the original data is technically challenging. Also, if the data had been transferred for review or early analysis, completely replacing it introduces the possibility that the new batch of data might include changes to the original values. The best approach, full or incremental deliveries, will depend on the entire data management process and analysis plan.

Typical problems

Programmers of the applications and data managers responsible for loading lab data have to plan for common occurrences such as:

- Mismatches of lab demographic data against CRF data
- Duplicate tests that may be true duplicates or separate retests
- Lab assessments of whether the result was normal

These will have to be addressed whether through the loading program or through the handling process.

Electronic lab files generally do have demographic data for a patient, but sometimes it does not match that of the data on the CRF! Each data management group must decide whether to ignore this data, use it during loading to identify possible discrepancies, or store it and cross-check the data later. Mismatches can mean that the data is being assigned to the wrong patient at the lab. Duplicate tests are frequently reported. Sometimes the result is inadvertently re-reported and sometimes the assay is repeated. Most labs will indicate a retest in the file, but this does not always work. Data management must decide how to handle retests: should all tests be stored or should previous or duplicate tests be removed? Lab files frequently flag values that are out of range. Some sponsors choose to ignore these values and recheck once the data has been loaded. Others may choose to load the information and still recheck.

Using loading applications

Loading is a kind of data entry and warrants a well-documented process. The lab data administrator or responsible data manager should log in the receipt of files or diskettes and check them for computer viruses. To provide documentation that the data was loaded, there should be a record of some kind as to the date the data was loaded, the amount of data loaded, and any problems encountered. (See Chapter 10 for further suggestions on data transfers.) Finally, like CRFs, the original lab data belong in some kind of archive, either paper or electronic.

Quality assurance

The processing of laboratory data should meet high standards, whether the data come in on a CRF or in an electronic file. The data management plan can be used to document any special handling or processing that applies only to lab data for a given study. For electronic data, a formal transfer specification should be required. This may be created by the lab or by the data management group but should be signed-off by both sides. On the sponsor's side, some kind of tracking must support the assumption that all the lab data has been completely and correctly loaded.

The quality of electronic data depends not only on the loading applications but also on the lab that sends the data. Not all labs have the technical support to consistently send files at the right time with the right data, and not all labs follow good data handling procedures. While clinical staff is typically responsible for auditing labs, data managers are sometimes involved. In particular, they can help check data handling and data correction procedures based on their experience as recipients of similar data.

SOPs for processing lab data

Normal SOPs for data entry cover the entry of lab data from CRFs. If there are no SOPs or guidelines governing the transfer in (or out) of data in general, a specific set of procedures should be developed for laboratory data loading. Normal discrepancy processing procedures can apply to both CRF and electronic data. Since review of lab data by data management may turn up possible safety problems, it is worth having some kind of policy, procedure, or guideline in place to define how such a concern should be handled.

Taking lab data seriously

Somehow, laboratory data seem to be the most problematic of all the data in a clinical study. The large volume of laboratory values common to many studies is certainly a key factor; the complexity of the interrelated tasks associated with the data is another. The volume and complexity can make it hard to pay careful attention to all that is going on with the data. However, data management cannot cut corners here because the data is critical to the study and subject to close scrutiny by many groups outside of data management as they assess the safety and efficacy of the treatment. Data management groups must allocate appropriate resources from the set up of the database right through the final transfer and study lock.

chapter nine

Collecting adverse event data

During clinical studies, patients always have undesirable experiences. These may or may not be related to the study drug or device. These experiences are known as adverse events (AEs) or adverse experiences and may be considered adverse effects or adverse drug reactions if there is a relation to the treatment. The strict definitions of what is an adverse event (AE), an unexpected AE, and a serious adverse event (SAE) are found in the Code of Federal Regulations (21 CFR), the European standards (EN), and International Standards (ISO). Data managers typically do not make judgments about what is an adverse event and what is a serious adverse event, but they do need to understand enough about the data to process and store them properly.

In many ways, adverse event data (AE data) is just like other clinical data. Such data is collected through case report forms (CRFs) or electronic screens and stored along with the other patient data in the database. However, certain aspects of AE data add two important tasks to the data management process: (1) the regular coding of the reported terms, and (2) the need to cross-check SAE reports in the data management system against those in the company's SAE system. Because both of these tasks can be made easier or harder by the way in which the AE data is collected and stored, we will look at collection first and then discuss coding and reconciliation.

Collecting AEs

People new to clinical trials may not realize that nearly all patients have some kind of AE during the course of the study. Remembering that the events do not actually have to be related to the treatment, the sites report everything from colds, to falls, to car accidents, to murder, as well as all the typical medical conditions that might be monitored by any doctor. The longer the study and the sicker the patient population for the trial, the more AEs there will be.

AE information for clinical trials can be grouped into three collection types or categories:

- Open AE reports
- Expected signs and systems
- SAE reports

Open AE reports do not prompt the investigator or patient for any specific problem. The event is reported either in the patient's own words or using the investigator's version of the patient's words. This is the most common way that AEs are reported during a clinical trial as the open format does not prejudice the investigator or patient in any particular direction. However, when a treatment has already shown a history of certain kinds of AEs, the clinical protocol may call for an assessment of the frequency and severity for those specific events during the course of the study. In this case, a list of these specific signs and/or symptoms may be used and the patient or investigator identifies which did in fact occur with a yes/no answer. In both types of collection, the investigator generally makes an assessment of the severity, relationship to the treatment, and action taken, as well as providing information on start and stop dates or whether the event is ongoing.

Either an expected sign or symptom or an open AE must be considered a SAE if it meets the regulatory criteria of: results in death, is life-threatening, requires inpatient hospitalization or prolongation of existing hospitalization, creates persistent or significant disability/incapacity, or is a congenital anomaly/birth defect. Any SAE requires the site to quickly report it directly to the responsible safety group (the sponsor's or contract research organization's [CRO's] as appropriate). In clinical trials, SAEs are also recorded with the rest of the patient data on CRFs or ECRFs.

While the open AEs and signs and symptom types of data will appear on different pages or screens, the data is similar enough that they can share similar structures (or even the same structure) for storage to allow for easy pooling of data. SAE information may be collected on the AE page or on a separate page as discussed below. There are also options to consider both for the content of these forms and on their positioning within the overall CRF booklet or study design.

AE forms

AE forms will collect a lot of data, including:

- The text used to describe the event
- Start dates (and possibly times)
- Stop dates (and possibly times) or an indicator that the event is continuing

- A variety of indicators including severity, frequency, relationship to drug, and action taken
- Additional comments or additional treatment/medication information

With so much data to collect, the fields take up a lot of space on the CRF, so much space, in fact, that many companies end up just having one or just a few AEs per page or screen. When only one AE appears on a page, it has the advantage that each AE can be monitored and collected as it resolves. When there are multiples on the page, all the AEs must be resolved before the page can be collected. Because AEs are often called for during interim analysis or for review by safety-monitoring committees, having the ability to collect all complete AEs easily can be a big work saver. Unfortunately, what saves work for data management, may create work for the sites and site monitors!

At some companies, the AE forms will have a box or question that asks: "Is this a serious adverse event?" and if it is, the site is instructed to fill in additional information on that page. At other companies, SAEs are always and only reported on separate forms. Companies should avoid having a site answer the question: "Is this a serious adverse event?" and then instructing them to *also* complete an SAE page. Having the same event appear on both an AE page and an SAE page can have unpleasant impact; there are bound to be discrepancies between the events when sites transcribe the reported term and other fields. Also, the groups reporting counts of AEs to the Food and Drug Administration (FDA) must always be aware of, and take into account, the "duplicate" reports.

Some companies opt to collect AEs at each visit. Other companies prefer to have the AEs in a "log" portion of the CRF. In the first case, the site asks the patient about AEs at each visit and fills in the form. The tricky question is what to do about events that are not resolved at the time of the visit. They should probably be marked as "continuing" but then at the next visit, does the original report have to be re-entered if it has resolved or are only new AEs recorded at that time? Input from all groups represented in the study team is needed to pin this down and determine how the data is to be analyzed and reported. This can be a daunting disadvantage. The main advantage is a powerful one: the AEs are monitored when the visit is monitored and are available to be entered in the database.

In the case of the log-type AE collection, the investigator still asks about AEs at each visit but they are all collected in one spot in the booklet or at one screen tab. For any AE that is ongoing, the site leaves off the resolution information until it does resolve. The only AEs marked as continuing should be those that are ongoing at study termination for that patient. This greatly simplifies analysis of the AEs but collection then becomes a problem as monitors will often leave the pages until the end instead of collecting them as they are resolved and monitored.

Data and database considerations

Except in the case of a signs and symptoms page, the reported AE term is a short free text. All of the usual problems of free text apply to these, including restrictions on the length of the field, misspellings in the term, and the use of abbreviations or special punctuation. These normal problems are made more serious by the fact that this text will be coded against an AE dictionary, and the coding process tends to be complicated by even minor variations in the text. (See the sections later in this chapter for more on AE coding.)

Most forms request start and stop dates (and possibly time) of the event. If an event is ongoing at the time of recording, companies will frequently have the site check a box for "continuing." Knowing when the event occurred helps the sponsor determine association with the study treatment. (For example, was the patient even on the drug at the time the event is recorded?) Unfortunately, in many studies, the time between visits is long enough that the patient may not exactly remember the exact dates for each event. The study designer and clinical group must determine whether the investigator and patient should make a good assumption and provide a fully complete date or whether a partial date can be accepted. These decisions must be made at the beginning of the study as they will determine the type of storage used for the dates and the kinds of cleaning checks performed.

Because the onset and resolution dates are so critical to analysis of the event, checks on these dates are critical. Clearly the resolution date should be after the onset date. But there are other checks as well: the protocol will usually give the period during which AEs are to be collected; for example, from screening to 30 days after drug termination. Dates must fall within this period (although many companies will never ask that any AE, regardless of when reported, be removed from study data). Checks against other dates in the study may also be required such as a comparison of the date of treatment discontinuation when the action taken for an AE is "treatment discontinuation."

If an event can occur more than once and be recorded (with different start and stop dates, of course) on the *same page or screen*, then some kind of information to differentiate the two events in the database will help in processing. A unique line number or sequence number, which may or may not appear on the CRF page, can solve this problem. Even when all the events are different, unique numbers on AE pages that have multiple reported events is particularly useful in writing queries to the sites.

AE reports include the investigator's record of the action taken in response to the event. Most frequently, the sponsor presents a coded list of possible actions. The study designer, database designer, and the investigator must be clear as to whether the question requires a single response or whether multiple actions are permitted. Storage methods will be very different if a single or multiples are an option.

As we noted in Chapter 2, an indicator box that says whether there were any AEs helps clarify if the page has been overlooked or if there are no data when a page comes in empty. But, as in all such cases, the question of "Any adverse events?" can cause some additional work in data cleaning and discrepancy management when the response is ambiguous. Data management must come up with guidelines for how to manage inconsistencies, such as an answer of "Yes" but there are no events listed, or an answer of "No" or blank when there are events on the page.

The regulatory requirements for reporting on AEs are quite high. The requirements apply not just on a study-by-study basis but rather on a larger scale of drug or device and may require summaries across studies conducted anywhere in the world. Because the reports must combine AEs across studies, it makes sense to standardize AE collection and storage from the beginning and to keep it consistent across studies over time.

Coding AE terms

To summarize AE terms, report on them, assess their frequency, and so on, analysts must group terms that are the same. "Headache," "mild headache," and "aching head" should all be counted as the same kind of event. This grouping or categorizing is done by matching (or coding) the reported AEs against a large codelist of AE terms, more commonly called a dictionary or thesaurus. In the past, coding specialists performed this coding to the thesaurus by hand. Now, nearly all firms use some sort of computerized, automatic matching called "autocoding." Data management, a safety group, or a specialized coding group may be wholly or partly responsible for tasks associated with running the autocoder and manually assigning codes to terms that do not match the dictionary automatically.

The autocoders all involve some level of text matching with or without special lexical transformations (see Chapter 23) so the coding process is heavily dependent on the text found in the AE reported term fields. To aid the coding process, some companies request that data management correct certain clear misspelling in reported terms, adjust abbreviations, and make other minor text changes to facilitate coding during data entry and review. This is usually done in the term field directly but the modified text may also be stored in a secondary field in order to keep it separate from the original reported term.

When a term cannot be coded because it is a combination of terms (e.g., "headache and nausea," which should be listed separately), data management may be asked to split the term themselves. While splitting may not be a problem, it is not clear whether all the data associated with each term (onset date, severity, etc.) apply equally to both terms. As the FDA becomes more vigilant regarding safety data, companies are becoming more conservative in handling safety data. The current trend is for data management to issue queries to the sites for all discrepancies or problems associated with AE data, including splitting terms.

Reconciling SAEs

SAEs from clinical trials and marketed products are supposed to be reported directly to a safety group or safety coordinator. Because of the detailed information related to the case of a serious event, and because of the reporting requirements, these safety groups frequently use a specialized system for the processing and management of SAE data. The SAE report (called a case) is entered in this system initially and updated as follow-up information becomes available. All reports to regulatory agencies are run from the case data in this system.

SAEs that take place during clinical trials should *also* come into the company with the rest of the patient's trial data. This version of the information is then entered separately into the clinical data management system. The clinical data management system is the source of SAE data to be used in analysis, reports, and new drug applications to regulatory agencies.

Before the end of the study, the SAE information in the safety system must be compared with that in the data management system to ensure that all SAEs were collected and reported properly in both systems. Data managers generally call this comparison process "reconciliation." Data management staff, when reconciling, look for:

- Cases found in the SAE system but not in the clinical data management (CDM) system
- Cases found in the CDM system but not in the SAE system
- Deaths reported in one but not the other, perhaps because of updates to the SAE report
- Cases where the basic data matched up but where there are differences, such as in onset date

This comparison of the cases is always a problem because of the different ways the information is collected in the two systems. The clinical data management system imposes a fair amount of structure on the event data. The patient and investigator information is well defined and consistent with other study data, there is age and sex information collected (separately) in the study, and the AE information is collected on an event-by-event basis with information associated with each reported problem. SAE systems impose less structure on a case. There may be patient and investigator ID information collected, but it may also be left blank, and the information about the event itself is collected as longer narrative text. This narrative text is then distilled into reportable and codeable terms by the safety group. Because of the different ways of reporting the words used to describe an event in the CDM system they may not be the same words used to describe the event in the SAE system. Even the coding methods or algorithms used by the two groups may not be the same!

Some differences detected during reconciliation may be obvious, but in some cases, the medical monitor working with someone from the safety group will have to determine whether an SAE in the data management system is close enough to that in the safety system to be considered the same. Data managers may be responsible for extracting and reviewing data but they should not be in charge of making decisions on medical concepts.

Methods for reconciliation

With all these difficulties and differences between the systems storing SAE data, most companies still rely on reports and a manual comparison to reconcile information. If the reporting tool being used has access to the underlying application (or database, such as Oracle) in both systems, it might be possible to do an initial match on some information, such as study ID, patient number, investigator, and a date. A manual comparison of the events can then assure that they are both complete and comparable.

Those companies attempting automatic reconciliation face great challenges. They must first identify which type of data is to be reconciled and then specify which fields to compare. Generally, only AEs cases or individual events termed "Serious" according to regulatory definitions are reconciled. As noted before, the wording of the reported terms might actually be different in the two systems, so it is not possible to match on those, but if the same coding dictionary is in use *and* both sets of terms have gone through coding, it is possible to match on the result of the coding (e.g., preferred term). The patient and protocol number must be consistent between the systems to make any connection at all. Clearly, there are many "ifs" before any automatic reconciliation is even possible.

Easing the reconciliation process

In an attempt to circumvent or at least ease the problem of reconciling cases, a few companies have designed processes in which the information is entered only once or a single source is used to enter data into both systems. For example, the appropriate CRF page is faxed in to the safety group for SAEs and it is *not* entered into the clinical database at all, but only into the safety system. In another example, a special SAE report form is used to enter the case into both systems separately. Note that in this latter case, there is still the problem of updates to the case, which then also have to be coordinated and performed in both systems.

Some companies have built or purchased systems to transfer SAE reports between data management systems and SAE systems. The technical problems are manageable: the database fields and structures in the source system (e.g., the clinical data management system) are mapped to those in the target system (e.g., the safety system). Because CDM underlying structures tend to be more flexible than those of safety systems, mapping is made easier if the CDM structures are carefully designed to match those of the safety system by:

- Collecting the same fields using the same data types
- Collecting all the data considered mandatory by the safety system
- Assuring that all codelists match
- Storing dates in compatible formats
- Using similar coding methods

Still, because of the underlying differences in the systems and different people collecting the data, there will be problems, and an expert review of each transferred case may be required. In general, the problems of case transfer tend to be less the technical issues than the issues of process or procedure that lead to differences between the data.

Quality assurance and quality control

The quality and accuracy of AE data is critical. In both paper based and electronic data capture systems, data management groups can help ensure quality by providing clear processes on handling the data, coding, and reconciling. For paper based studies, many companies perform 100% data audits on the AE terms and related information to check the accuracy of transcription.

When a company uses standard AE forms, there are likely to be standard structures. Given how critical these structures are to reporting and reconciliation, guidelines should dictate that these cannot be changed without a high-level review. Standards generally result in improved quality across studies.

SOPs for AE data

Normal data entry guidelines should sufficiently cover the entry of AE data, although there may be special procedures that outline permitted and required changes to reported terms to assist the coding process. If changes are permitted, they must be carefully documented in department or study specific guidelines. In addition, the SOPs should require that the changes be recorded in the data management system audit trail, meaning that they will made after initial entry, typically by more experienced staff.

SOPs for reconciliation will touch on several groups besides data management and so should be coordinated and signed-off by everyone involved in the process. The procedures should clearly spell out responsibilities for providing database listings, safety systems listings, discrepancy reports, site queries, data updates, and so forth. SOPs or study specific guidelines should also spell out when reconciliation is to take place. Traditionally, reconciliation has only been done after all the data has been entered, before study lock. As we see a higher expectation that companies be aware of possible safety problems with their treatments, some companies are going toward more frequent, even monthly, SAE reconciliation, with final reconciliation again at study lock. No matter when reconciliation takes place, evidence of the reconciliation must be in the data management or clinical files. Ideally a medical monitor signs-off on the final reconciliation, if not the intermediate ones.

Most SOPs and guidelines governing coding are presented in Chapter 23, but it should be noted here that a sign-off on coding is often required as part of the procedures on study lock. This is true whether data management is performing most of the coding and manual assignments or if an outside group is doing the work. Sometimes the medical monitor is given a list of all unique terms encountered in the study and their codes to review and sign. In other cases, the medical monitor will review only those terms that required manual assignments (i.e., they did not autocode). The requirements should be clearly spelled out in SOPs or study specific documents such as the data management plan.

Impact on data management

While AE data is, in many ways, like any other data collected during a clinical trial, it is critical to the evaluation of the safety and efficacy of the treatment. In particular, AEs add coding of reported terms and reconciling of SAEs to the data management process of a study. Both of these tasks tend to be particularly active as close of the study nears. Reconciling, in particular, may not be possible earlier in the course of the study, and even if performed earlier, will have to be repeated at the end of the study. The effect then, of AE data as a whole, can be to impact the close of a study. Data managers may not be able to change this, but they can be aware of it and plan for it. When sign-off on coding and SAE reconciliation is required to lock a study, data management must notify the medical monitor or responsible party that his or her attention will be required in order to avoid surprises and/or delays in lock.

chapter ten

Creating reports and transferring data

Data management is frequently responsible for producing reports or listings of study data for internal staff and management. Some of these reports are standard representations of the data, which are run over and over on current datasets. Other reports are ad hoc reports, that is, the format and content is requested by a user of the data for infrequent or one-time use. Users of standard or ad hoc reports may be data management staff, clinical research staff for medical review, management to monitor progress, auditors, and so on. The level of effort devoted to the creation of these reports depends on the users and the use to which they will put the report.

Transfers of data to internal or external groups may also fall to data management. For example, a small company may require the transfer of data to an external statistician for early or final analysis. In other cases, the transfer may be to a partner company or to a client (as in the case of a contract research organization [CRO]). Because transfers of data nearly always involve safety and efficacy data for storage or analysis, the level of effort devoted to a transfer must be much higher than that for most reports.

The layout of a report or the format of a transfer file is not its most important attribute; the content is. Users must know where the data come from, how it was selected, and when it was extracted. Ideally, all of this information is included in or otherwise evident in all reports and transfers created by data management. Then, of course, the contents must actually reflect what was specified and this is where testing and validation come in.

Specifying the contents

The specification of what data is to be included in a report or transfer can be simplified by asking: "From where," "Exactly what," and "When?"

99

From where?

The study or studies from which the data is extracted identifies where the data come from. The study or protocol information should appear, at least, in the header or notes of a report and should be firmly associated with the data (e.g., via a file name) when the data come from a single protocol. If the report or transfer contains data from across studies, then the study identifiers should appear with the associated data as a variable. While the inclusion of this information seems obvious, it is often left out of ad hoc reports under the assumption that the report is being run over a single set of data anyway. In the case of transfers, it is a common problem when multiple datasets are shipped as a group and are identified in some cover memo and then the identifier is lost when the datasets are split up or reorganized.

Exactly What?

The selection criteria information used to extract the data is critical to its interpretation. This is especially true if the variables or fields used in the selection criteria are not actually included in the report or transfer. For example, if a listing contains only data from male patients, the patient's gender might not actually appear as a column in the listing but would impact any conclusions drawn from the data.

The selection criteria should not disappear from the final report or data. For reports, the information might appear as text in a report header, title, or footnotes. Including selection criteria information in transfers is more difficult because transfer files frequently do not have titles, headers, or other places to store comments pertaining to the file. To be totally clear, the data fields used in the selection might be included as variables or columns in a listing or transfer even if they appear to provide redundant information. Another option is to include the information in a transfer file (described further later) that accompanies a data transfer.

In addition to the explicit selection criteria, there are usually some hidden or implicit criteria or conditions applied to the data. These hidden selection criteria frequently have to do with the "cleanliness" of the data. A simple selection of *all* the demographic data in the database, for example, could well select data that has only gone through first-pass entry and still contains transcription errors. It would also very likely contain data that has not yet been cleaned and may not even have had edit checks run over it. In the case of electronic data capture systems, a complete extract of that data would likely include data that has not yet been monitored! The specification of every report, listing, or transfer should clearly state what data is acceptable for the particular use.

When?

The date the selection of the data was made may or may not be the same as the date the report or transfer was performed. There will often be a lag if the reporting tool or program being used makes a "snapshot" or copy of the data for its work or if the tool is using a data set transferred from another group or company. In these cases, the extraction or copy of the data copy will be made, but the report will only follow a few days later. While this is not usually a serious problem, it regularly causes confusion in sponsor interactions with CROs. The sponsor will look at the date the report was run and forget that the data was extracted quite a while ago and may not reflect true, current status. Ideally, the date associated with the report or transfer will reflect the day the data was *selected* rather than the day the report was run.

Standard and ad hoc reports

Some reports can be well defined and are used over and over either within the conduct of a study or across studies. Examples of this kind of report include patient accrual, lists of outstanding discrepancies, and data dumps of lab data. These reports can be considered "standard" reports. Other reports are used infrequently or are created to deal with a particular data problem or need. These reports are frequently called ad hoc reports. Ad hoc reports are built to answer an immediate question or need and are typically not designed to work in other situations and so are quickly developed. The level of effort put into the creation of standard reports tends to be higher since the intent is to make them generally useful. In both cases, however, careful thought must be given to how the report will be used to determine the level of validation necessary.

If either a standard or ad hoc report is to be used to evaluate, or make a decision concerning, the safety and efficacy of a treatment, it should be subject to validation. If a report is to be used for mainly administrative, tracking, or data management review purposes, it should still be properly designed and tested but would not need a full level of validation (see below). Some reports may be used in ways that do not clearly fall one way or the other and require a judgment call to determine the extent of validation necessary. A good rule of thumb is to assess the risk of getting it wrong. If a report fails to list some specific data, what would the outcome be without that data? Would the information be caught in another way or at another time? Would it make any difference to the outcome of the trial or the analysis of the data? If the risk is low, the level of validation can be low or lower than for critical reports and transfers.

Even when validation is needed, the level or extent of the validation effort should not exceed that needed to build the report. One possible validation approach for important, standard reports would be to require the following:

- A short (<1 page) specification of what the report will contain or present (specification)
- A description of the tool or tools to be used and the logic used in selecting data for the report (technical documentation)
- Sample results or output (technical documentation)
- A summary of test data used and output of tests run (testing)
- If appropriate, a short description of how to use the report or make it run and any limitations or assumptions (user documentation)
- A restriction on changes or a change control process

All standard reports would have to meet these requirements. The more critical the report, the more effort is put into the validation effort. Obviously, the output of the validation would be stored in an appropriate file (see Chapter 20 for more details).

Note that the validation effort for these reports does *not* include validation on the tool or software package being used to create the report. Any validation deemed necessary by the company and the associated general testing of such tools should have taken place at the time of installation. The validation effort for reports focuses on the correct or appropriate use of the tool or application.

Contrast the validation effort for important reports against the process for creating ad hoc reports. Ad hoc reports might only require a brief specification and result of testing before being used on production data. The testing might even take place on "real" data, but someone would confirm (by hand) that the appropriate data was included and that the output was correct. While the creators of ad hoc reports may still follow good process (including asking for specifications and checking the results), few companies require that documentation on ad hoc reports be kept on file and they permit changes as needed.

Data transfers

Transfers of data is different from reports in that the data is copied and sent elsewhere (either within, or external to, the company) to be analyzed, reviewed, and reported on. Transfers of data nearly always involve or include some safety and efficacy data. Because of this, data transfers should be guided by Good Clinical Practice, and data management must see beyond the simple creation of an electronic file, which is just the first step of the transfer *process*.

The transfer process involves creation of the transfer file(s) using a validated program or application, checking correct and complete selection of data, moving the file(s) to the transfer medium, and preparing transfer documentation. Two techniques for improving and documenting the process are the use of transfer checklists and transfer metrics.

Transfer checklists

Even if the transfer is a one-time occurrence, a checklist of the steps needed to produce it helps ensure that nothing is overlooked. If the transfer is repeated during the course of a study or studies, the checklist is essential to ensure consistency and completeness at each transfer. The checklist should be created *before* the very first transfer, even if all the steps are not known until a few test runs have been completed: the act of documenting before doing helps point out undefined areas and allows cross-checks to be built in from the start. Figure 10.1 illustrates the steps that might be in a checklist for transfer from a PC to a CD.

Just creating the checklist is usually not enough to make sure all the steps are followed. Even the most conscientious data manager may overlook a step. Guidelines that require printing the checklist and initialing each step on completion usually help ensure that all steps are followed. The checklist provides excellent documentation for the transfer and can be filed with a copy of the transferred data.

Transfer metrics

Transfer metrics are numbers that help verify that the data was completely extracted to the transfer file. Exactly which metrics will be useful for any given transfer will depend on the format and number of the transfer files and on the type of data being transferred. Some of the common transfer metrics include:

Activity	Initial When Complete
Create transfer directory on the PC	
Run program to extract data	
Review metrics generated by the extraction program	
Start a metrics file for the receiving group; copy in values	
Compress all transfer files	
Add compressed file sizes to metrics file	
Print out metrics file	
Copy all files (including metrics file) to CD; make two copies	
Check both copies on another PC for readability	
Store one copy; send the other CD along with a paper copy of metrics file	

CD sent by: _____ Date: _____

Figure 10.1 An example of a transfer process checklist. This example assumes the data is copied to a PC and is then transferred to a CD.

- Number of files
- File sizes
- Number of patients per file
- Number of records per patient
- Number of variables or fields

Some companies also create a checksum (a number generated by an algorithm that is unique to the contents of the file) for each file that can help detect corruption of the contents of the file.

Data managers review these metrics once the transfer files have been created to get a sense of whether the transfer program put the correct data in the file. This is useful even if the data manager does not know exactly how many patients or records to expect. The user receiving the transfer can also benefit from these same numbers to determine if all the data was properly made available on receipt. Because the numbers are useful at the receiving end also, they can be sent along with the transfer in an information or metrics file. The metrics file can also provide a convenient place to document the selection or extraction criteria, the date the data was extracted, and any other assumptions or special conditions in effect at the time the transfer file was created.

Review of printed reports and presentations

At some companies, data managers are involved in quality control of printed reports created by other groups. This might include tables in the study report, slides to be presented to upper-level management, or data to be included in articles. They are asked to manually check any raw data values (not statistical results, of course) before they are made public or presented. They look for appropriate selection of variables (for example, those in standard units rather than the raw values from the case report form) and scan the data to see if it fits with their knowledge of the study. The idea here is that data managers are most familiar with the data and so can most easily check its accuracy.

For small companies, this may make sense but even then processes must be in place to assure that:

- The request is placed with enough lead time to carry it out.
- The data is in fact updated if a data manager sees a problem.
- That data is rechecked if the report or presentation is substantially changed.

SOPs for reports and transfers

At a minimum, companies should have specific standard operating procedures and/or guidelines that spell out the validation requirement for reports and the quality control or verification of transfers. The procedures need to address documentation and testing requirements for the different kinds of data contained in the reports or transfers and the different uses to which they are put.

Putting in the Effort

In theory, companies will allocate resources and effort to meet quality and regulatory requirements, but practically, that does not always happen. If a company has to choose between putting an effort into validating reports and verifying and checking transfers, it should choose to put the effort into transfers. As just about everyone who has been the recipient of CRO or lab data knows, when a transfer goes wrong or is missing data it causes no end of trouble. And often, that trouble goes further "downstream" as the data is used by programmers and statisticians. Backing it all up and getting a fresh, correct transfer irritates everyone involved and has a serious impact on timelines.

Companies should still take the validation of critical and standard reports seriously. Validation does have value by itself in improving the quality and ease of use of reports, not just value in meeting regulatory expectations. That being said, we do still see overkill in validation efforts undertaken for low-risk reports. Companies must set reasonable requirements and allow some variation in how the requirements are met to avoid making validation more work than writing the application.

chapter eleven

Locking studies

After the last patient's data has been collected from the sites, the race is on to close and "lock" the study. Once a study has been locked, the final analysis can be made and conclusions drawn. Because there is usually high pressure to make those analyses (and related decisions) as soon as possible, companies frequently keep track of "time to database lock" and work constantly to minimize that time. The pressure to quickly lock a database for analysis comes up against a long list of time-consuming tasks that need to be performed first. The list involves many individual steps, including: collecting the final data, resolving outstanding queries, reconciling against other databases, and performing final quality control (QC).

Once these tasks are performed and someone signs off on them, the study is considered locked. (That is, no data value will be changed.) The data is now considered ready for analysis. Statisticians and upper management will begin to draw conclusions from the data under the assurance that it is unlikely to change: unlikely to change, perhaps, but it is not uncommon to detect problems or find missing data after a study lock. If there are enough changes or the changes are serious enough, the study will be unlocked. There are usually specific conditions that can lead to unlocking a database, restrictions on what can be changed during the time it is unlocked, and requirements that must be met before it can be relocked.

In this chapter we look at the most common steps performed for a study lock and discuss unlocking and relocking before addressing some ways in which the time to study lock can be reduced.

Final data and queries

Before a study can be locked, it must contain all the clinical data generated by the study. The data, first and foremost, is the original data from the patient reported on case report forms (CRFs) or through electronic case report forms (eCRFs), but there is other data as well: corrections from the sites, calculated values, codes for reported terms, and data from labs. Any of this final data may generate discrepancies that will require resolution before study lock.

To account for all the original data, data management uses tracking information to ensure that all expected CRF pages have been received; there should be no missing pages. In addition, the lab data administrator will check that all laboratory data was loaded and that any other electronic loads are complete. Once in the central database, this data will go through the cleaning process, which may generate discrepancies. As the final data comes in, the final calculated values also must be derived. Discrepancies raised by calculated values are usually traced back to problems with the reported data and may have to go back to the site.

All reported terms (such as adverse events [AEs] and medications) must be coded and any changes to terms that come in as corrections must also be rerun. When a term cannot be coded, a query may have to be sent to the site, but close to study lock some companies will permit a medical monitor or clinical research associate (CRA) to make limited corrections to the reported term to allow it to be coded. Just to be sure everything is in a final, coded state, many companies rerun coding at the end of the study to catch cases where the assigned code changed due to a change in the dictionary or synonyms table or cases were the term was changed but the code did not receive an update.

Resolutions for the new discrepancies, as well as those still outstanding from earlier in the study, are also required for completeness. Generally, all outstanding queries must have a resolution, even if the resolution is that a value is not available, before a study can be locked. Getting these last resolutions from the site can hold up the entire closure process, so CRAs frequently get involved in calling or visiting the sites to speed corrections. Because of the difficulties and time pressures at the end of the study, companies may choose not to pursue noncritical values at this stage of the data handling. Ideally, the list of critical values will have been identified at the start of the study in the data management plan and can be referred to when facing getting a resolution from an uncooperative site right before study lock.

Some companies call the point at which the last CRF comes in from the site "soft lock" or "freeze." Other companies wait until the last query resolution is in to declare a "soft lock." In either case, this is the point at which the real work of assuring quality begins. The data is not locked yet because there may still be changes to the data that come out of the lock activities, such as database audits, but the number of changes is expected to be small. The data is in a near-final state.

Final QC

The quality of the data will affect the quality of the analyses performed on the data. At the close of the study, there is a particularly strong emphasis on checking on the quality of the data that is about to be handed over to a biostatistics group. Because there is, or should be, a high barrier to getting a study unlocked, it is worth making an effort to check the data thoroughly.

All kinds of review of the data help provide assurance as to its quality and correctness, but study closure checklists frequently include these specific kinds of checks:

- Audits of the database
- Summary reviews of the data
- Reconciliation against other systems

Accuracy audits

Data transcribed from a CRF or other source into the database is usually checked for accuracy through a database audit. Data managers compare data in the database against the CRF and any associated correction forms. Many companies still perform the audit near the close of the study to determine an error rate. Unfortunately, if a late audit does detect problems, correcting them will prove challenging and time consuming. A more efficient approach is to perform audits early and, if appropriate, repeatedly, to catch systematic problems. Then, at the close of the study, the data to be audited would be either the final data only or fields identified as critical or in some way risky to the study. This can be especially useful when the audit plan calls for a 100% audit of key fields. In this case, the audit of the key fields can begin as patients are considered "clean," that is, without any outstanding discrepancies. (For a further discussion of audits see Chapter 5.)

One of the big advantages of electronic data capture (EDC) systems is not having to audit the database looking for transcription or entry errors. However, even for electronic data capture (EDC) studies, sponsors should consider a check of all changes to data that were made in response to queries. This check can be performed on an ongoing basis or as part of QC checks at study lock. Experience has shown us that edits made to correct errors often introduce new errors. This is likely to be as true for site staff as it is for data entry or data management staff. Not all EDC systems (and the processes associated with using those systems) would support such a review, but it can be considered.

Summary review

There are certain kinds of cleaning or discrepancy checks that are better performed near the close of a study when the data is more complete. These include listing reviews, summary reports, and simple analyses of the data as a whole. The goal is to detect unusual values that stand out in the context of a set of data but that might otherwise pass cleaning rules or other discrepancy identification methods.

A listing review of text fields is a good example of how trained humans pick up inconsistencies that cannot be programmed into edit checks. Data managers may review listings of text fields to check for nonsensical words that are introduced because entry operators are focusing on what they see rather than the meaning of a phrase. A separate listing review by CRAs is often required for study lock. The CRAs may notice nonsensical phrases and the like, but, more importantly, they may find problems with protocol compliance. For example, they may review medications and find some listed that are not permitted by the protocol. Or, they may find medications listed in the medical history section. They may even find serious safety problems listed in comments associated with lab results or AE reports.

Humans are very good at detecting patterns or unusual values. Listing reviews of numeric values may also work for smaller studies to detect unusual values or outliers. For large studies, summary reports created from ad hoc queries or simple statistics performed on the data can identify unusual patterns or outliers by looking at the:

- Number of records or values per patient
- Highest, lowest, and mean for numeric values
- Distribution of values for coded fields (e.g., how many of each code)
- Amount of missing data

These summary reviews can be run by data management staff but in some companies, clinical programmers will look at the data using SAS.

Graphs of lab and efficacy data or other simple displays or analyses can also can identify possible problems with units, decimal places, and different methods of data collection that might not otherwise be caught by simple cleaning checks. These will probably come out of the programming or statistical group. In the end, the best review of the data is to run the planned analysis programs on the data even before it is locked. The goal is to have no surprises when the final programs run!

Reconciling

In the best case, clinical data is stored in a single location and extracted for review or analysis as needed. However, in the setting of a drug or device trial, it is not unusual for the data to be stored in more than one location, and for very good reasons. When this is true, reconciliation may be necessary to ensure consistency between the systems.

The most common reconciliation with external systems is for serious adverse events (SAEs). Data on SAEs are typically stored in both the clinical data management system (CDM) and also in a separate SAE system. When reconciling at study close, data management staff look for:

- Cases found in the SAE system but not in the CDM system
- Events found in the CDM system but not in the SAE system
- Deaths reported in one but not the other — perhaps because of updates to the SAE report
- Instances where the basic data matched up but where there are differences, such as in onset date

See Chapter 9 for further discussion of AEs and the reconciliation process.

Another common source of duplicate storage occurs when a trial uses an interactive voice response system (IVRS) to randomize the patient or assign a treatment via a kit number. The IVRS will store responses and the assigned treatment group in its database and the CRF or eCRF design may also require that the assignment be recorded. Reconciliation between the CRF and the IVRS is a very good idea; in a trial of any size, expect that some of the information will not match. In fact, it is very important to know if the IVRS assigned one kit number but the site provided a patient with a different kit number (for whatever reason).

Companies have also found themselves reconciling against paper in cases where sites are asked to provide additional information to the study monitor for AEs that are appearing more frequently than expected. For example a medical monitor may note that certain events were occurring more than expected, "rash" for example, and send letters to the sites to get more information on those events. These would not be CRFs. In filling out the additional information, the site may report medications that were not provided on the concomitant medication forms or they may provide information about the AE that does not match that reported on the AE forms. In this case, there is no other option than to manually cross-check the sources of information (additional info form and database) and notify the site if there is a discrepancy.

Locking and unlocking

The exact checklist of procedures to follow before study can be locked comes from a data management standard operating procedure (SOP) or study specific requirements documented in the data management plan. Once all of the items in the study lock list have been completed, permission to lock the database is obtained. Typically, a manager reviews the closure procedures and associated results and signs off on the list. Permission is then obtained from the clinical group and biostatistics to show that everyone is in agreement that the data is as complete and accurate as possible at that point. (This dated lock form should *always* be filed in the study file.) The data management group then physically locks the study against changes. The idea is that the study stays locked, but unforeseen problems with the data or unexpected new data can force a temporary unlocking of the database.

Locking

Different data management systems provide different means of accomplishing the physical lock. At the very least, this involves removing permissions on the data so that only a privileged user (such as the database administrator) could make modifications. In many systems, this removal of permissions must be done manually, sometimes on a user-by-user basis. Other CDM systems have ways of tagging or flagging the data as being locked. The tag typically accomplishes the same thing as removal of permissions (i.e., modifications to the data is prevented) but has the advantage of being more easily set than a manual removal of permissions for each user or user group.

When permissions are removed for locking, it usually means that the entire study must be locked at the same time because it generally is not possible to remove permissions from individual patients or from subsets of the data. The tagging method, on the other hand, may allow subsets of the data to be locked as they are processed. If a company has a strong need or desire to lock subsets of data (e.g., when data is sent out in incremental sets, or if patients are being cleaned individually over a long period of time), data managers may have to set up a tagging method by adding special lock fields to the data and processes to set and check those lock tags.

Unlocking

Once the study is locked and data analysis begins, it is not uncommon to find problems with the data that require corrections. (This is particularly true if final quality control does not include summary reviews of the data or draft runs of the analysis programs.) New information regarding AE data found during site close-out or site audits may also require edits to the data. A request to unlock the study usually requires review of detailed reasons by higher level management before the database administrator removes the locks. Unless the changes required are extensive, the database administrator will grant permissions to very few users. Appropriate quality control, review, and approval will again be required to relock the study. Many companies require that the lock checklist be used to relock a study.

Time to study lock

Time to study lock is one of the key data management metrics. It is also the one metric that gets a lot of attention from other groups. To understand time to study lock we need to understand the start point. If a company is measuring time to lock from the time of the last patient visit, then the time can be quite long. That data must be monitored, the CRFs brought in, the data entered, verified, and checked. Discrepancies on that data must be registered, reviewed, and possibly sent for resolution. There is a lot of variability introduced here due to travel schedule and site availability. Measuring time to study lock this way does not account for a study's number of sites and staffing. Time to lock measured from last query resolved is more consistent from study to study.

Note that some EDC system vendors will say that it is possible to lock studies in their systems one day after the last patient is in. Most data management groups will disagree with this claim. Discrepancies are raised (and many resolved) during entry of the data at the site and the data is also available for review immediately, but most companies still require that that data be monitored. After monitoring (or in parallel), all the other activities of a study lock have to take place, except for database audits. Because they do not require a database audit and because site communications are sped up, EDC systems *do* lock faster than paper based studies, just not immediately.

After study lock

The lock of a database is such an important milestone in a study that staff will push hard to meet the deadline and then breathe a sigh of relief because the work is done. Unfortunately, it may not be quite done at that point. Before everyone moves on to new projects and forgets details, managers should allocate time to make sure the study documentation is complete and to record feedback from the study.

Most data management groups try to keep the study file fairly current, but it is nearly impossible for it be totally current at all times. It is a very good idea to have a study file audit shortly after lock. The lead data manager should check the file to ensure that all required materials and documents are present. Documents should be the most recent version and have current signatures if required. The list of who worked on a study and what they did should reflect the final status. This is also a good time to add "notes to file" to record any unusual circumstances or data related to the study.

Very few companies schedule feedback meetings after a study lock. Unfortunately, people forget details and problems very quickly as they move on to new studies and problems may be repeated. Right after lock is a great time to review the CRF or eCRF for fields that caused an unusual amount of trouble. Those fields, or modules, should be modified, if possible, not just reused for the next study. This is also a good time to review the metrics from the study such as:

- Total number of pages (perhaps average time to enter)
- Number of staff needed for the study
- Total number of discrepancies
- The percentage of discrepancies resolved in house
- The percentage of discrepancies from sites requiring a data change
- The top ten types of discrepancies
- Average time to resolve queries
- Time from last query in to study lock

The more information a data management group has from a locked study, the more accurately the forecasts and estimates for the next study will be.

Quality assurance

The most important thing about study closure procedures is to make sure no step is missed. The easiest way to assure a complete and consistent process is to follow a closure checklist and require a physical signoff. The best way to assure that the data is really ready to analyze, is to analyze it in its near final form before the lock.

SOPs for study lock

An SOP for study lock and unlock should be considered high priority. In some cases, the list of steps to be taken before lock will appear in the SOP. In other cases, the SOP will simply require that a study specific checklist be used, and perhaps set minimum requirements for that list. As noted before, a high-level manager should be responsible for final signature for both lock and unlock.

Reducing time to study lock

The best way to reduce the time needed to lock a study is to avoid leaving things until the end. This not only helps ensure that the study is closed soon after the last query resolution is received but also improves the quality of the data by detecting problems soon after they have been introduced. Companies should consider the following approaches to data management tasks that can shorten time to study close:

- Enter data as soon as possible after it is received. Data on paper does not move the process along.
- Run cleaning procedures throughout the study as data is collected so that the queries go out early. Toward the end of the study, the outstanding queries should be only those pertaining to recently received data.
- Identify missing CRF pages and lab data by knowing what is expected. Use tracking systems.
- Code AEs and medications frequently.
- Reconcile SAEs periodically throughout the study. Since AE and SAE data often come in late in the study (e.g., AEs may be ongoing), get listings from the safety system early so you know what to expect.
- Begin to audit data against the CRF (for paper based trials) early in the study to detect systematic problems. Continue to audit as the study proceeds to monitor quality.
- Open the study documentation at the start of the study and make an effort to keep it updated as the study progresses.

For tasks that cannot be performed before the end of the study, the best that can be done is to understand the amount of effort involved to complete them. At this critical point in the study timeline, data management should provide as good an estimate as possible for the amount of time required to carry out a task properly, since other groups depend on the outcome and the deliverable. These other groups will be planning also and will not appreciate major adjustments to their schedules!

part two

Necessary infrastructure

This section of the book focuses on the infrastructure necessary to perform data management work in a regulated environment. Without the appropriate infrastructure in place, a data management group cannot perform the work consistently and may not be complying with Food and Drug Administration regulations. The first three chapters on standard operating procedures, training, and security specifically address regulations requiring written procedures, qualified staff, and restricted access to clinical data.

The fourth chapter in this grouping addresses the data management interaction with contract research organizations (CROs). While this interaction is not as explicitly regulated and rarely audited, it does constitute a critical piece of infrastructure. Nearly all companies will use CROs for data management at some point, sometimes even exclusively.

chapter twelve

Standard operating procedures and guidelines

At nearly every training course, workshop, or seminar on standard operating procedures (SOPs) the question floating around in many people's minds is: "Why do I need SOPs," or "Do I *really* have to have SOPs?" Sorry, but the answer is "Yes." International Conference on Harmonization (ICH) guidelines and Food and Drug Administration (FDA) regulations explicitly require SOPs. The ICH document "E6 Good Clinical Practice: Consolidated Guidance" states:

> 5.1.1 — The sponsor is responsible for implementing and maintaining quality assurance and quality control systems with written SOPs to ensure that trials are conducted and data is generated, documented (recorded), and reported in compliance with the protocol, GCP, and the applicable regulatory requirement(s).

Other FDA regulations and guidance documents, including 21 CFR 11, also specifically refer to the FDA's expectation of certain SOPs governing particular processes.

There is really no way around having SOPs. There are still some very interesting questions, though, about SOPs and SOPs for data management, in particular. This chapter will look at what SOPs are, what procedures should be standardized (that is, what is the list of common SOPs), how to develop those SOPs, and how to assure and document compliance with SOPs.

What is an SOP?

Standard procedures are standard procedures, but they do appear under a variety of names: standard operating procedures (SOPs), departmental operating procedures (DOPs), guidelines, working practice documents

(WPDs), company user manuals, and so on. While the philosophy behind the way these documents are written and maintained might be different, an auditor could ask to see them all to understand how tasks are carried out and would expect that all standard procedures be adhered to.

The different names for standard procedures reflect the level of detail they contain and the target audience. The procedures that apply company-wide to all trials tend to be called SOPs. If the company is large and has many data management departments, they may have procedures that are specific to their department or country. These are often called DOPs. While it is not universally true, SOPs and DOPs tend to be written at a high level to outline required tasks, sign-offs, and checks performed without specifying details of the systems used, or the individual steps needed to carry out a particular task. It is more common to put details specific to systems, and steps detailed enough to be used as a training guide, in other documents. This kind of document might be called a "Work Instruction" or "Guideline."

When a company uses the multilevel approach, the SOP-level procedures reflect company philosophy, regardless of underlying systems or with only light reference to those systems. They are written with the expectation that modifications will be infrequent. The specifics on how to implement those SOPs in a particular environment are found in one or more associated guidelines or work instructions. Company specific user manuals can provide yet further detail of how to use a particular software application to support the procedures. Guidelines and manuals are likely to be more frequently updated, in particular, as new versions of associated software systems are implemented. Here is an example of text from three different levels of procedure documents:

- **SOP:** "All data from case report forms (CRFs) will be double-entered."
- **DOP or Guideline:** "Data will be double entered using the third party arbitration feature of the clinical data management (CDM) computer system. The first and second passes are to be performed by two independent entry operators."
- **User Manual:** "To begin third party arbitration after the data has been entered twice, open the Enter menu and select 'Arbitration' from the drop-down list."

Whether the detail is found in an SOP or in a guideline, the effect should be the same. There should be standard procedures covering all key elements of the conduct of the study. These procedures should provide enough detail to ensure they are consistently carried out, without providing so much detail as to end up with violations of the procedure because of normal variations in working. Also, each procedure should include a description of appropriate materials (forms, documents, checklists) that must be produced to document that the procedure was in fact carried out. This is the evidence needed to show the SOPs are being complied with.

SOPs for data management

Those SOPs specific data management would need to cover all the elements of the data management process. Because the process is reflected in the data management plan (described in Chapter 1, or the entire first section of this book), those can be used as a starting point for a list of SOPs. Appendix B lists a comprehensive set of topics to be covered by SOPs that apply to data management. This list was compiled from a wide variety of sources and covers both specific SOPs mentioned in regulatory publications and SOPs that have become expected, or industry standard. It is important to note that the list in Appendix B is a list of topics, not SOP titles. Some topics may naturally be combined into a single SOP.

In addition to SOPs specific to data management tasks, the FDA lists recommended SOPs in its guidance on "Computerized Systems Used in Clinical Trials." In small companies, the data management group may need to make sure these are covered. In larger companies, these are generally covered by information technology SOPs or in SOPs developed for validation groups. In any case, it pays to be sure that some group somewhere in the company has procedures for:

- System Setup/Installation
- System Maintenance
- Data Backup, Recovery, and Contingency Plans
- Security and Account Maintenance
- Change Control

The list in Appendix B is quite a long list of procedures for new data management groups to be faced with. Unfortunately, there is no example set of SOPs available as a starting point, and most companies keep their standard-procedure documents confidential. Experienced staff can use their prior exposure to and experience with SOPs as a place to start, but companies, company philosophies, and company needs differ so much that the procedures have to be written mostly from scratch.

Creating standard procedures

In small companies or new groups, data managers are sometimes faced with creating a large set of procedures from scratch. (At established companies, they are more likely to revise existing SOPs over time.) Both emerging and established companies have to deal with the need to write new procedures and guidelines covering new systems and applications. When starting from scratch, small companies have to come up with a vision and prioritize. When writing for a new system, all companies have to juggle the need to have something in place when it goes into production with the problem of perhaps not fully understanding the new system and its features.

Starting from scratch

When faced with the task of creating a whole set of SOPs and guidelines, it helps to start with a vision and a plan. The data management team begins by coming up with a list of the procedures to implement, an index of sorts. In reviewing the list, the group then provides a brief description of what the procedure will cover and whether it will be general or detailed. Because it is impractical to write and implement all the proceedures at once, the next step is to prioritize.

Since a group faced with the task of creating a whole set of procedures is likely to be preparing for an imminent study or perhaps the close of a single study, the best way to prioritize may be to begin with the SOPs necessary to complete imminent tasks. When getting ready to set up a new study, the group may prioritize the areas needed at the start of the study and those most critical to ensure quality. This priority list might include:

- Study setup and test
- CRF tracking and workflow
- Entering data
- Collecting and coding adverse events

If the group is also faced with the imminent installation of a new system to support data management, an SOP on system validation, or at least a standard validation plan outline, is a must. An important part of a validation packet is information that is collected at the time the system is first installed and configured. It is hard to collect that information without knowing what will be required!

Once the group has decided on a list with priorities, it reviews the company template for SOPs. (This assumes there is one; templates are available online and in books for groups who have none.) Because the description of the procedure and how it should be carried out forms the heart of the document, that is a better place to start than defining "Responsibilities" or "Definitions." Those will eventually fall out of the description of the procedure. The description includes what prerequisites the task has and where the task begins and ends. It lists any input into the procedure as well as any output. If there is a specific workflow to follow, that is laid out here also. An SOP should answer the questions: "Who?" "What?" "Where?" "When?" and "How?"

Quality professionals generally suggest that the people who actually perform the work be involved in writing or defining the procedure description, though ultimate authority in making it "standard" lies with managers. This often puts managers and the staff members who do the work in conflict. Those performing the work will write a procedure that reflects how it is being done now, or in the case of a new data management group, how those people did the work at a previous company. The managers, on the other hand, are often looking to write a procedure to reflect how they think the work *should* be performed. Managers must be very careful not to let the procedure become too theoretical. It is not a good idea to set up a theoretically good procedure and then find that the group disagrees strongly, has never seen anything like it, or simply cannot carry it out the way it is written.

As the group defines the procedure, they should keep asking themselves: "How will we know people are following this procedure?" For any procedure important enough to warrant an SOP, it is worth having some kind of output, outcome, or other documentation to show that procedure has actually been carried out as defined in the procedure (more on this below).

Procedures for new CDM systems

As we will see in the chapters on system implementation and validation later in this book, SOPs and guidelines are integral parts of bringing in a new software system. They must be in place (and still applicable) when a new system goes into production use. Any existing procedures and guidelines must be reviewed to make sure they still apply and are accurate. The problem is that internal staff may not be sure enough of how the new system works to provide the details. This lack of experience presents less of a problem for SOPs written at a general procedure level than for detailed guidelines, manuals, or work instructions where precision counts.

At the time a system goes into production, the people with the most experience are those who have been responsible for the implementation, the users that tested the system, and those who have performed the pilot (if any). Reviewers of existing SOPs and writers of new SOPs and guidelines should tap into the knowledge and experience of those groups. After installation, the implementation team (who has received early training) can provide enough information to create a draft procedure. If testing is performed before a pilot, the testers can provide feedback on some of the details. Ideally, by using these two sources, the procedure writers will be able to make a good draft available for the pilot or initial study that is to be brought into production in the new system.

One of the goals of the first study should be to try out the draft procedure. The team commits to working according to the draft procedure as much as possible and allots time in the middle or at the end of the study for reviewing and updating the procedure. If the first study is an actual, not "pretend" study, then care must be taken to document in the data management plan and/or study file that the procedures used for certain tasks were draft versions. The goal should be to have a solid set or procedure approved before any more (or perhaps, more realistically, *many* more) studies go into production.

Complying with standard procedures

Standard procedures do no good at all, and a considerable amount of harm, if they are not followed. The two best ways of assuring they are followed is to make sure that everyone knows what the procedures say and to make sure the procedures stay relevant. Even if everyone is following a procedure, but there is no evidence in the form of a document or output to prove it, it does not count. When writing SOPs, data management groups must be sure that the evidence is built in.

Training on SOPs

Training is the first step in making sure staff members know the procedures. For new employees, this usually means SOP training soon after they begin and before they are allowed to perform work on production studies. Smaller companies provide this training one on one; larger companies hold frequent SOP training sessions. Note that contractors and other temporary employees must go through the same process if they are to be involved in carrying out some or all of a particular procedure! In addition, as noted in Chapter 12, documentation of the training must go in the employees' training files.

Despite the fact that SOP training for new hires is a standard practice, most people admit that new employees cannot be expected to remember the details of the SOPs after a one-time training. At a minimum, they need to have ready access to them. This used to take the form of providing a paper copy of the SOP and guideline set for each employee, but keeping paper copies current has always been a challenge. More recently, SOPs and guidelines are made available on company intranet Web sites. The Web sites have the advantage that they always have the most current copy of the SOPs and can support additional notes, comments, templates, and examples.

Training will also need to take place whenever an SOP is revised. Usually, the manager or trainer will focus on the difference or new procedures in the revised document. However, trainers often find it more practical to just review the entire procedure and this has the added benefit of giving everyone a refresher course on what they should be doing. Because it can take days or weeks to train everyone on revisions, most companies have notification systems that build in the lag time needed for training before the SOP actually becomes effective. That is, everyone is notified that a revision has been approved and is ready for training, but that new procedure does not become effective (meaning people have to follow it) until sometime after the approval date to allow everyone to complete training.

Designing for compliance

Even training and ready access still cannot guarantee compliance. The best guarantee of compliance is to write SOPs and guidelines that actually can be followed. The following characteristics, found in an SOP, will often lead to noncompliance:

- Too-tight timeframes
  Be sure to allow enough time for the natural and appropriate workflow. Can you really get a signature within one day? Do you really

have to have sign off on all edit check specifications before *any* programming can begin? Perhaps it is sufficient to have sign-off before edit checks can be run in a production environment?

- Overspecified details
  Do notations really have to be done in green ink or is any pen color other than black acceptable? Does a batch transmittal form always have to have initials by the clinical assistant who opens the mail or can it just be whoever opens the mail?
- Documentation produced after the fact
  Asking for burdensome documentation after a particular task has been completed is asking for trouble. This is especially true if the work has to be performed after study lock. It is much better to require only documentation that fits naturally into the process and actually adds value to the procedure rather than trying to document something that happened in the past.
- Overuse of the words "require" and "will include"
  If something is "required" by an SOP, it had better be there during an audit. Do not require documentation, forms, or output if it is not *always* part of the process. If something does not always apply, then "recommend" it or specify it as "may include."

If you write a procedure and it turns out not to work in practice, record this outcome (also known as a "deviation") either according to company policy or as a study specific note to file. If the same deviations happen over and over, arrange for a revision of the procedure as soon as possible. Not following a standard procedure may actually be viewed by an auditor as worse than not having a written procedure!

Proving compliance

As many people in the field will say, "No SOP, no GCP" or "If it wasn't documented, it wasn't done." If a company has great SOPs but there is no consistent evidence that the procedures were followed, then for all intents and purposes, the procedure wasn't followed. Now, this statement is taken a bit to the extreme because there is often intrinsic evidence that a procedure was followed and explicit evidence is not always required. Still, whenever a group is working on an SOP, they should ask themselves what the proof would be if an auditor came in and said, "Prove to me you do this consistently." For SOPs guiding particularly important processes, such as serious adverse event reconciliation or locking a database, it is a good idea to have clear documentation that all required procedures were followed.

The best evidence of compliance is something that is used in carrying out the procedure specified in the SOP (an SOP "tool"), or something that is naturally produced as output when carrying out that procedure. The idea should be that whatever you file as evidence of compliance should also be helping you carry out the procedure. For example, when an SOP has many steps or steps that take place with a time lag (such as might be found in study lock procedures) consider using a checklist. That checklist not only provides great evidence that the steps were carried out, but also helps keep staff members from inadvertently missing a step. As an example of a natural output from a procedure consider using the annotated CRF as evidence that the designer followed the procedures for SOP on database setup. That annotated CRF is hugely valuable to anyone working with the database and is not "extra" documentation provided to show how a database was designed. (A printout of the database structures completes the picture and can provide a quality control step if compared to the annotated CRF.)

Less useful but generally acceptable types of evidence are the common sign-off forms found associated with many procedures in data management. These usually have a title such as "Study Lock Approvals" followed by a list of people, identified by position, who have to sign off to approve a process in advance or to attest to the fact that the procedure was carried out. These are really not tools, they are just evidence. In using them, we have to rely on the idea that the signers were diligent in making sure all the necessary steps were, in fact, carried out.

SOPs on SOPs

Yes, there should be an SOP on SOPs! This procedure is usually developed at the corporate level and typically would contain references to the required sections of an SOP or point to a company template. Ideally, the SOP on SOPs would also give some guidance as to what goes into SOPs as opposed to guidelines or work instructions as well as what level of detail should be provided. Finally, the SOP should require review of each SOP within a period of time (typically on the order of one and a half to two years) from the time it becomes active.

SOP work never ends

Let's imagine that a data management group has all the SOPs in place that they feel are necessary. About that time, if not before, they are going to start at the beginning and review each of them. Procedures change so the SOPs that govern them must be updated regularly. Systems change and SOPs have to be reviewed to see if the software has forced a change to the documented procedures. Regulations change and FDA guidance documents change; SOPs may need to be updated. Industry practices also change over time and it is worth asking if a procedure perfectly acceptable five years ago is now falling out of the mainstream of data management groups. Or, perhaps a new procedure has shown itself to be effective. SOPs are definitely not static. Most auditors expect SOPs to be reviewed at least every two years or so, and they may well be suspicious if a document has not changed in more than two years.

Many companies have written the requirements into company-wide policies and procedures mandating that SOPs be reviewed on a regular basis. Once SOPs are in place, data managers are understandably reluctant to open them up again. The best thing to do is to plow ahead with the review and attempt to keep minds open to the idea that this is a chance to improve the process and revisit the tools or other compliance evidence to make the SOP work better for the data manager.

chapter thirteen

Training

Just as standard operating procedures (SOPs) are required as infrastructure, so is training of staff, or perhaps more significantly, documentation of that training. Training is listed explicitly in the regulations, as we see in the International Conference on Harmonization (ICH) document "E6 Good Clinical Practice: Consolidated Guidance" which states: "2.8 — Each individual involved in conducting a trial should be qualified by education, training, and experience to perform his or her respective task(s)." 21 CFR 11 echoes this in section 11.10, which states that the procedures and controls related to maintaining electronic records will include: "(i) Determination that persons who develop, maintain, or use electronic record/ electronic signature systems have the education, training, and experience to perform their assigned tasks."

Perhaps even more interesting than the text of the actual regulations are the comments from the FDA found in the introduction to 21 CFR 11. On pages 13450–13451 and 13464, the agency responds at length to comments sent in by the industry during the review phase of the rule. They use the responses to questions regarding training requirements to emphasize that the FDA believes training specific to the task is required and they conclude by saying:

> The relevant education, training, and experience of each individual involved in developing, maintaining, or using electronic records/submissions must be documented. However, no specific examinations or credentials for these individuals are required by the rule.

Because data managers use clinical data management systems (CDM), they are creating and maintaining electronic records that will be used in submissions. They will have to document their training and experience. This chapter will discuss approaches to satisfying these training requirements, identify some common problems in setting up training, and touch on approaches to address those problems.

Who gets trained on what?

The place to start with training is to decide who is trained on what. Many companies have a matrix or spreadsheet of positions in the company and the SOPs that people holding those positions must be trained on. While SOP training is important (see Chapter 12), an SOP list is the bare minimum for identifying the training staff members must have. Training on an SOP will not provide training on the company's data management system, specific workflow, or study specific procedures. In addition, the use of the title or position to select the SOPs often leads to overtraining on SOPs for procedures some people will never perform and do not need to know. A better approach is to define all the kinds of training available and link that training to roles rather than positions.

Note in Figure 13.1 an example of a training matrix where roles identify the kinds of training that staff members must have in each of four different areas. The training table has columns not just for SOPs but also for CDM system training, pertinent guidelines, study specific training, and practice or tests. The SOP training applies if there is an SOP that covers the role or task in question. The system training refers to any training required for using the CDM system or other software. The guidelines column lists all the guidelines that apply. The "Study Specific" column indicates that there is study specific training required for *each* particular study. For example, someone joining a study already in progress to help with discrepancy management should be trained on the study's edit checks and on any study specific discrepancy handling instructions before he or she begins work. Finally, the test column indicates whether there is a test, practice, or work

Role	1. SOPs on:	2. CDM System	3. Guidelines	4. Study Specific?	Test Required?
First pass entry	Data entry CRF workflow	Entry menu	"Handling Pages with No Identifier" "Data Entry Guidelines"	Yes	Entry test
Second pass entry	Data entry CRF workflow	Entry menu verification features	"Handling Pages with No Identifier" "Data Entry Guidelines"	Yes	Verification Test
Discrepancy-resolution	Discrepancies	Discrepancy menu	"Discrepancy Management"	Yes	No, work review only
CRF designer	Designing CRFs	N/A	"Managing CRF Files"	No	No, work review only

Figure 13.1 An example of a training matrix where roles identify the kinds of training staff members must have in each of four different areas. The final column indicates whether a formal test is required to qualify to do the work.

review required before the person can perform the task on production or "live" data. There may be a practice data entry that is reviewed before a new entry operator can begin work but for discrepancy management there may be no test if a reviewer just checks that person's work for a specified period of time.

While nearly all companies provide training on data management topics in general, they do not all yet specifically require study specific training. Study specific training for clinical staff has been required for quite some time and attention is now moving to provide it for data management. There is growing recognition that even studies involving the same treatment, performed at the same company, using the same data management system, still have differences worth pointing out. These differences will be small in companies with strong standards and in those cases the training may be minimal. In emerging companies, these differences may be quite large and well worth spending an hour on!

A final note on roles: by training based on the role a person plays within data management or even within a study, it should be clear that temporary workers and contractors will get the same training as permanent employees. Training for contractors is often neglected but should not be. They do the work, they need the training.

How to train

Only large companies have training groups, and even then those groups often focus on company-wide training. They may train on corporate SOPs, good clinical practice in general, and other topics that pertain beyond data management. A data management group that is large enough and lucky enough may have a data management trainer, but it is extremely common for data management to be responsible for its own training.

If a data management group is relatively small with low turnover, one-on-one training may be the most efficient approach. While many small groups assign new staff members to a buddy or mentor for training, this leads to wide variability in the quality of training. A better approach is for, one person in the group who is both interested in and good at training to be the designated trainer. If the group is growing, periodic formal training sessions may become worthwhile. In this case, the quality of the training will probably improve and be more consistent, but there are always issues about holding the classes when they are needed. As Web-based training becomes more available, even to smaller companies, it may provide the consistency of training found lacking in mentor-based training, support part-time trainers, and make courses available as they are needed.

Training records

One of the first things an auditor will ask for is training records. That usually sets off a flurry of activity as the manager of the group requests the files from whoever "owns" them. If the training records are housed centrally, they will be easy to retrieve but are less likely to be current and complete. If the training records are maintained by the employees, they are more likely to be complete, but harder to find. Both of these approaches have their pros and cons, and each company must explicitly weigh them to make a decision. The solution may be Web-based training records, which, at this writing are not yet widespread; but, given the fast spread of Web-based training mentioned above (where records, however, are often still kept on paper), having employees and trainers maintain the records on a company intranet may soon address this problem. After deciding where the records are to be kept, companies should also be clear exactly what should go in those records.

A typical training binder will have tabs or dividers for the person's résumé or curriculum vitae (CV), company-wide SOP training, and then group-specific SOP, guideline, and other training. Let us look at each of these tabs to define useful contents.

Because the regulations require that each person be qualified by "education, training, and experience," training records need to record the "education" and "experience" part as well as specific training. A résumé or CV is typically used to satisfy this requirement and it is placed prominently at the beginning of the training file. The CV should be fairly current. That is, employees should be instructed to review and update their CVs yearly. Many companies ask that the CV reflect the person's current position in the company.

Education is not only formal schooling. It also includes seminars, workshops, and other relevant courses that employees attend. These are valuable additions to an employee's education and should be noted in the training files. With the current emphasis on training in the industry, nearly all organizers of external courses or seminars will print certificates of participation for those who stayed through the end of the course. Employees should be encouraged to keep a copy of these for their own files and a copy (or original) in the training binder. Even conferences add to a person's experience and education and, therefore, add value to the training records. Conferences can be listed separately or added to the employee's résumé. If there is no separate tab for external training, it should be placed behind the CV.

Now we address the company and data management specific training sections that cover SOPs and guidelines. Many companies advocate the approach of filing only a training sign-off sheet and no materials actually related to the training. That is, SOPs, guidelines, training slides, practice sheets, and so forth do *not* appear in the training binder. The idea is that when given to an auditor, the additional material not only makes it more difficult to assess training, it also provides too much insight into details of processes. On the other hand, some companies *do* like to see more information about training, such as outlines or agendas, along with the sign-off form. In both cases, the trainee, trainer, and date trained should be readily apparent.

Just as many companies are only now considering how to train on study specific tasks, they are also considering how to *file* records for such training. There are good arguments for filing study specific training in the study files and there are also good arguments for filing that material in the training binders. At this time, there does not yet seem to be a consensus or trend, so either is acceptable.

The same effort that goes into training files for employees should go into training files for temporary workers and contractors. If an auditor requests a list of names of people who worked on a study, that auditor is then free to ask for training records for any of those people. Responding that one or another of those names belongs to a past contractor will not be acceptable. Always maintain training records for everyone who worked on a study. If training files are maintained by employees, collect the files when the employee leaves the group or company. The manager must always be able to pull those records as well as those for current employees during an audit.

SOPs on training

Not all companies have SOPs on training, but they usually do have very specific instructions on maintaining training documentation. If there is no company policy in place, each data management group can set up a practice of having training plans for new employees. The training plan can cover the three areas of training: SOPs, department guidelines, and system training as recommended in this chapter. Study specific training can be enforced through data management plans or requirements for the study files.

Allotting time for training

Probably the biggest mistake smaller companies make is not allotting time for training. They specifically hire experienced people and then expect each person to jump in and begin work. After all, that person has done this work before. That person may have done the work before, and he or she may even have used the same clinical data management system but not done the work at the company in question. As we see in the first part of this book, there are many options on how to perform clinical data management and also how to make use of clinical data management systems. Each person needs to understand how the task is to be performed in each group's unique combination of procedures and system configuration. This takes time and may mean the new hire sits around a bit while waiting for training or review of work, but it is well worth the investment for all involved. State up front to each new hire (and the group) that new staff members should not expect to do production work for the first week or two (or even more). When the expectation is clear, no one will feel the new person is "wasting time."

chapter fourteen

Controlling access and security

The Food and Drug Administration (FDA) is very concerned, and rightly so, about the quality and integrity of data associated with clinical trials. In 21 CFR 11, and in guidance documents, the agency repeats the term, "authenticity, integrity, and confidentiality of electronic records" frequently to get the point across. The regulation is clear; §11.10 requires controls and procedures including: "(d) Limiting system access to authorized individuals," and "(g) Use of authority checks to ensure that only authorized individuals can use the system, electronically sign a record, access the operation or computer system input or output device, alter a record, or perform the operation at hand."

Limiting access (who can get in) is achieved through proper account management. Authority checks (who can do what) are set up via access control or access rights. Account management deals with assigning and maintaining user names and passwords. Access control defines how those users are given access to particular features of the clinical data management system (CDM) and how and when that access is revoked. Good account management and access control has to be achieved through a combination of the features of the CDM (or electronic data capture [EDC]) system and procedures to make sure the features are used properly and to fill in gaps in the system's abilities.

Account management

Accounts that are used to access CDM systems provide the user with varying degrees of power, or control, over data stored in the system. When the account permits the user to enter, modify, or delete data in electronic records, the user name and password together constitute one kind of electronic signature. It is not the kind of signature that is the equivalent of a handwritten signature (such as the principal investigator signature for electronic case report forms [eCRF] in EDC) but rather is the kind of signature that makes the change to

133

the data attributable to a particular person. All data management systems automatically associate the person that is responsible for the entry or change with the data, usually through the user name. By thinking of the user name and password as the way to make actions on the data attributable, it is easier to put procedures into place that govern the user name and password in compliance with 21 CFR 11. The user name must uniquely identify a person and the combination of user name and password constitute a signature.

User names

Saying "User names must uniquely identify a person" sounds simple enough and most data management and EDC systems enforce unique account names, but there are some important, real-life situations to consider. For example, if the user name associated with a common actual name (e.g., "jsmith" for Jane Smith) is removed when a person leaves the group or the company, then the possibility exists that that account name would be reused some time in the future (i.e., when John Smith joins the group). In reviewing the data at a later time, it would then not be possible to immediately tell which person entered a particular record without referring to the dates of employment and the dates the record was created. It is best, therefore, to leave all account names in the system to prevent their reuse. When that person leaves, access permissions are removed but the account name remains to prevent reuse.

Since most systems store not only the user name but also the full name of the person using that account (thereby making the association of user name and person), permanently retaining the account also keeps the connection to the actual person. If a system does not do this automatically, the connection must be retained through some paper method. In fact, many data management groups keep a paper account record of the person's full name, signature, initials, and user name when a new account is created. The need to keep the connection to a real name brings up one more common problem: having two people with the same name working at the same time.

This is not the same case that we just considered. In that case, the user name may be reused but the first person was "Jane Smith" and the second person coming along later was "John Smith." In this example, we have people with the same name, both "Jane Smith," for example, working in the group at the same time. Because the system enforces unique user names, one of user names may be "jsmith" and the other may be "jsmith2." Recording the owners of those names as both "Jane Smith" would probably not be considered sufficient identification for a serious audit. When tracking user names, either on paper or electronically, record either the middle initial or a birth date or some other information to differentiate the two. This same differentiation probably has to be carried over to training records, signatures on documents, initials on actions performed, and so forth. This is a bother for the individuals involved but the idea of "attribution," that is, exactly who did what, is important in the eyes of the FDA.

Passwords

The password in combination with the user name is what makes the attribution work. It is the signature of the person doing the work that says, "Yes, I performed this action." Most companies in the industry are aware of good password procedures and implement them at the corporate level for access to networks. Standard practices include:

- Only the user, not the administrator, knows the password.
- The password has a minimum length (generally eight characters these days but six may still be acceptable).
- The password must be changed on a regular basis (definitely less than a year, probably less than six months) and cannot be immediately reused.
- Many companies also require at least one character in passwords that is not a letter, or that the passwords not appear in a dictionary.
- No one should do work while signed in as another person. That can be construed as falsification should the data come into question.

These procedures comply with the FDA's recommendations (found in the responses to comments to 21 CFR 11) that recommend enforcing procedures to make it less likely that a password could be compromised.

While information technology (IT) groups regularly enforce these standards for the company network, not all data management system administrators configure their applications the same way. A surprising number of companies, when audited, do *not* require regular password changes, nor do they enforce minimum lengths. A bit of digging has also turned up cases where employees change their passwords repeatedly when they expire to get back to their "favorites." In the same comments section of the regulation, the FDA says, "Although FDA agrees that employee honesty cannot be ensured by requiring it in a regulation, the presence of strong accountability and responsibility policies is necessary to ensure that employees understand the importance of maintaining the integrity of electronic records and signatures." Some groups try to make clear to their employees (temporary as well as permanent) the importance of good password control by requiring them to sign a statement acknowledging that they understand the seriousness of not adhering to company policies, but many still do not truly understand the underlying intent of the rules it is hard for managers to detect poor password maintenance.

Account time-outs

Another often-neglected situation is that of employees walking away from their computer to get coffee. If they are logged on at that point, someone else could sit down and access the data. This is clearly not desirable as the comments section of the rule states: "The agency's concern here is the possibility that, if the person leaves the workstation, someone else could access the workstation (or other computer device used to execute the signing) and impersonate the legitimate signer by entering an identification code or password." The FDA recommends an automatic disconnect or locking of the screen so that the user has to sign on again to continue. At some companies, this is a network setting; at others it is a setting of the data management application. In either case, such controls should be in place and the idle-time setting, the number of minutes after which the systems locks, should not be set too high or it is of no value. New technology should help in the future as there are already devices that will lock the computer activity when the user, who is wearing or carrying a signal device, moves a given distance away from the computer.

Access control

For the purposes of this chapter, access control is the combination of systems and procedures that define what access rights or permissions users have to the clinical data in a CDM system. (Access rights for EDC systems are a bit different, but the information in this chapter can easily be extended to cover those as well.) Data management systems all have support for granting and revoking access to studies but the systems available may not meet all the needs of a data management group. In that case, procedures, with appropriate controls, should be put in place to fill the gaps. No matter how it is accomplished, systems and procedures should be able to answer the questions: "Who had access to a particular study, when did they have access, and what were they allowed to do?"

How to grant access

It is fairly standard in the industry at the time of this writing to grant access based on the concept of "roles." A role is a database term that describes what users will do in the software system. Will they enter data? Will they build a database? Will they manage discrepancies? The roles are created first, and then the role is granted access or permissions to studies. Often systems are set up so that the roles are granted access automatically at study creation based on a default specification. Users are added to the role or granted the role when they need to perform the activity.

The advantages to this approach are mostly from easy maintenance. The system administrator sets up the roles and decides on the appropriate permissions just once. Then, as users are added, they are assigned whatever role they need. When users leave or there is a change in the tasks they perform, they are removed from or added to a new role as appropriate. This works very well when roles are clearly defined and people who perform a role typically perform that role across all active studies. That is, everyone assigned to the "ENTRY" role can enter data across all studies. If, in fact, they are not *supposed* to do entry in a particular study because that is not their project, the restriction is enforced not in the system but through good practice.

Unfortunately, if a data management group does want to restrict access on a study-by-study basis, the administrator may have to make a role for each study. That is, now there is not just an "ENTRY" role but a role called "ENTRY_ABC01" that defines the permissions for entry work in study "ABC01." When the study is created, each necessary role is created and users are assigned to that role. This provides a great deal more control and also allows the administrator to ask for evidence of study specific training before the user is added to the role for that study. If the data management system has the study specific roles built in automatically, so much the better.

If, however, there are several different kinds of roles that are defined by the company implementing the system for each study, then the number of roles starts to become a problem in itself. If that is the case, groups should at least consider going back to the old way of doing things and assign access to users individually. The administrator will just grant the individual access to features and data as appropriate for the tasks that one person is to perform for any particular study. There is more work to be done in this case when studies are set up or locked or when a user leaves the group, but the specificity of control may well be worth the extra work.

No matter how the granting and revoking of access is accomplished, it should still be possible to answer the question of "Who worked on study ABC01?"

Who had access?

Auditors inspecting data management groups usually want to know, "Who had access to this study?" or they may phrase it, "Who worked on this study?" They are also either implying or explicitly asking, "And what did they do?" They don't often ask, "And during which time did these people have access?" but the question may arise should it be necessary to look at actual data and audit trails — something all of us hope will never happen at companies we work with! Nonetheless, it is worth asking ourselves how we would answer these questions.

Many data management groups keep paper lists of people who worked on a particular study along with their roles. Of course, whenever a process is manual, it is prone to be forgotten or delayed so it is much better if this information can come out of the data management system itself. The problem with data management systems as they are now is that they can easily produce current lists that answer the question, "Who has access right now?" but many (or even all of them) do not keep a history of access. That is, they cannot answer the question "Who had access last January?" If a person is removed from a role, the information that that particular account did have access to in the past is lost.

This has led many data management groups to start tracking access on their own, independent of the data management system. This tracking may be on paper, in an Excel spreadsheet, or in a database application, but however it is accomplished, it is done to ensure that answers to the questions of who worked on a study and what did that person do. Again, any process that is manual is prone to being forgotten so not only do they have to set up tracking, but they also have to build in checks to make sure that the tracking information is kept, at least most of the time!

SOPs and guidelines for accounts

Most companies have IT policies or standard operating procedures (SOPs) on account maintenance. A simple SOP or work instruction on account maintenance specifically for CDM systems would probably suffice to cover security and access. For EDC systems, procedures specific to managing site passwords and accounts, and in particular the account and signature of the principal investigator, are critical if data management is in charge of administering these.

Taking security seriously

The FDA takes secure access to the data seriously; data management groups should do the same. All data management groups should be able to show that they take appropriate measures to control accounts, maintain passwords, and that they can identify who performed what actions on the data, even if the study locked years ago. That being said, it does fall on every person to maintain his or her account according to company policies and procedures.

chapter fifteen

Working with CROs

The International Conference on Harmonization (ICH) document "E6 Good Clinical Practice: Consolidated Guidance" defines a Contract Research Organization (CRO) concisely as, "A person or an organization (commercial, academic, or other) contracted by the sponsor to perform one or more of a sponsor's trial-related duties and functions." CROs can perform many, if not all, of the tasks associated with the development of a drug, including developing drug compounds, conducting toxicology studies, carrying out Phase I to Phase IV clinical trials, producing a submission, and many more. Larger CROs may have the resources to provide any of these services, but more typically, a CRO will specialize in a few particular areas. Data management groups will have the most contact with CROs conducting clinical trials rather than those involved with drug development, for example.

A biopharmaceutical or device manufacturer chooses to use a CRO for a variety of reasons. Small and emerging companies frequently do not have the resources and expertise in house for all of the drug development tasks so top management makes a decision as to which kinds of expertise will be hired in and which will be contracted out. They may have a plan that will bring that expertise in house as the company grows. Larger companies turn to CROs to deal with changing capacity or for expertise in new areas of development. Even the best planning cannot possibly assure that there will be a steady and even flow of work in the drug development process, and CROs can help with the sudden need for extra capacity in a particular function. If a larger company is thinking of moving into a new area of research, management may choose to start with a CRO for the same reasons small companies use them: they can provide expertise until a need for in-house staff is well established.

Both the ICH documents and Food and Drug Administration regulations discuss the transfer of obligations of the sponsor to a CRO. They both state explicitly that regulations apply to CROs as much as they do to sponsors, *but, the sponsor is still legally liable for the data.* The ICH in E6 says: "5.2.1 — A sponsor may transfer any or all of the sponsor's trial-related duties and functions to a CRO, but the ultimate responsibility for the quality and integrity of the trial data always resides with the sponsor." In this chapter, we will discuss how to work with CROs to assure that data is processed in compliance with regulations and results in datasets that meet the sponsor's standards for its own data.

The CRO myth

It is a myth that using a CRO means the sponsor offloads all of the work involved in the project or that portion of the project contracted out. Contracting with a CRO to carry out an entire clinical trial or perform only data management tasks *does not* mean that the sponsor's data management group will have nothing to do with the study! It is only through close involvement with the study from the time of study setup, throughout study conduct, and through database lock and final transfer that a sponsor can feel confident about the quality of the data associated with the study.

It is by establishing a base knowledge of the CRO's compliance with regulations and industry standards that the relationship gets under way. This baseline is established via an audit of the CRO. Then, for each project, both sides must clearly define their responsibilities so that no critical data management step is overlooked. To really understand the data and data quality, the sponsor liaison must stay closely involved in the project through ongoing review of materials, oversight of milestones, and constant discussions about the handling of problem data.

Auditing CROs

A sponsor is ultimately responsible for the quality and integrity of the data coming from a CRO. It is generally accepted in the industry that a key component of accepting that responsibility is to audit the CRO before, or at least around the time of, beginning substantial work with that CRO. Sometimes a company will have the resources to maintain an audit group who will review a CRO's procedures in all areas of interest to the sponsor. This should include someone with data management experience if the CRO will conduct some or all of the data management functions for a study. In smaller companies, or when special expertise is required, data management may be asked to designate an auditor (in house or contracted in) to look specifically at data management functions at that CRO.

Auditing usually involves a review of written policies and procedures as well as interviews with CRO staff. Often, the auditor will work off a checklist or question list so that no key items are forgotten. By reviewing documents and talking with staff, the auditor gets an idea of whether the CRO performs up to industry standards and complies with regulations. Needless to say, if required to review data management practices in detail, the auditor must be very experienced in the field of data management and understand acceptable variations in practices.

After the audit, the auditor will write an audit report and highlight any significant findings, both good and bad. The auditor must be careful to differentiate between noncompliance with regulations and variations in practices. In the first case, immediate action would be expected and the CRO should have a detailed remediation plan with timelines. In the latter case, the sponsor may have a different opinion about what is "best practice" in a particular area but the CRO may still be using a fully acceptable approach. When this comes up, and the sponsor wants to continue to work with the CRO, the companies will usually work together to formulate a plan or compromise specific to the study.

It is wise to follow up on serious negative findings in a relatively short timeframe with another visit or some other means of checking compliance. For a successful audit, no repeat visit has to be scheduled, but note that the results of *any* audit have a shelf life. Because the industry is changing and because management and staff changes are to be expected at any company, sponsors should plan to re-audit CROs every two to three years, or sooner if some other change at the CRO warrants it.

Defining responsibilities

One of the most important measures a company can take to get a study and a CRO interaction off to a good start is to explicitly define the responsibilities of each of the partners. It is not enough to say that the CRO will be responsible for "data management." Who will create the case report form (CRF), track enrollment, reconcile serious adverse events (SAEs), code adverse events (AEs), review summary data, and so forth? The explicit list of responsibilities should be agreed upon even before the contract is signed. It should be worked out during the bid phase so that all CRO bids are on roughly equal terms. This also helps prevent "out of scope" charges when the CRO bills for tasks it had not figured into the original bid. A sample responsibility matrix can be found in Appendix C.

Oversight and interaction

Oversight of the project by the sponsor's data management staff or data management liaison starts as soon as the contract begins. Interactions should continue on a regular basis throughout the conduct of the study and into the study lock phase. The more time the sponsor puts into the study, the more the sponsor will gain from the study and the better chance of high quality data. That should be the key for the sponsor: high quality data.

Study startup

If the sponsor is not developing the CRF, the CRO's CRF or eCRF must be carefully reviewed, just as an internal one would be. In particular, the CRF should be consistent with, or reflect experience from, previous studies in the same area. The final sign-off for the CRF should come from both sides: the sponsor's team to indicate the CRF meets its requirements and the CRO side to indicate that the CRF design can be successfully translated to a database in their system.

Every CRO study should have a data management plan (DMP). This can come from the sponsor but is more likely to be written by the CRO's data management group. As discussed in Chapter 1, the DMP should cover all the data management tasks for a study. In the case of a CRO/sponsor relationship, the DMP should make clear whose procedures are to be followed for a particular task and to clearly identify points at which data or responsibility passes from one side to the other. The sponsor must review and approve the data management plan of a CRO and must be current on all the amendments that take place during the course of the study.

The following procedures may appear in the data management plan or as separate documents. In either case, the sponsor should review and approve documents and procedures related to:

- Data entry conventions
- Data management self evident corrections
- Study specific discrepancy handling instructions
- Receiving and managing lab data
- Coding conventions including study specific coding queries
- SAE reconciliation workflow
- Data validation plan (including all edit checks, manual reviews, and summary reviews)

The review of these documents and procedures, sending the feedback to the CRO, and then checking that comments have been incorporated appropriately is a time-intensive job. Sponsors should allot an appropriate amount of time during the study start-up phase to do all this. *It is the sponsor's responsibility to provide feedback and approval in a timely manner.*

Data management groups (both on the sponsor and on the CRO side) vary as to whether they expect an annotated CRF from the CRO to be reviewed by the sponsor. This may seem inappropriate since the sponsor may not even be familiar with the CRO's com system. However, as we saw in Chapter 3 a database from a CRF can be implemented in more than one way. Actual experience has shown sponsors that a review of the annotated CRF can turn up misunderstandings about the data to be collected before it is too late and too far into the study. Some time put in up front can prevent serious problems at transfer time or at lock.

That brings up the question of transfers. The CRO and sponsor together must define not only how the data is to be formatted for transfer (e.g., what the data sets or tables should look like) but also how often that data is to be transferred. This information goes into the DMP or into a separate transfer specification. As we will see below, a single transfer at the end of a study is never a good idea.

Study conduct

Once patient data begin to come in to the CRO questions will arise. The sponsor's data management liaison must be available to answer these questions. The best practice is for the study team, both CRO and sponsor staff, to meet weekly to discuss issues and deal with special problems. While clinical teams often schedule these meetings as a matter of course, it is critical for data management to be there also and to be there for most of the meeting. While listening to clinical and site-specific problems, data managers often pick up on plans that will impact the data or data management. It is the liaison's job to identify these issues and develop a plan together with the CRO's data management team for handling the problem data or special circumstance.

Receiving a data transfer at the end of a study or once before lock is usually not advisable unless the study is quite small and of short duration. Early and regular data transfers (or some other kind of access to the data) allow the sponsor to check the quality. While a sponsor should *never* re-program all the edit checks to run on the transferred data just to be sure that they were done properly at the CRO, a review of the data through simple summary statistics or line listings can identify places where new edit checks are needed, where CRFs need to be changed, and where sites need additional instructions. This review is frequently performed by data management, but it may fall on clinical staff as resources are available.

The sponsor and the CRO must agree on a procedure for communicating manually identified discrepancies uncovered by these reviews to the CRO's data management team. The sponsor will also want feedback on whether those discrepancies have been issued to sites or whether they need not be because the CRO has other information. This brings up two important points:

1. The sponsor reviewing data should not issue duplicates to automatic checks manually. That is, if the sponsor sees an empty field in the transferred dataset and knows there is an edit check to validate this field, no manual discrepancy should be issued. The sponsor's staff must trust that the CRO has performed the work unless there is evidence otherwise.
2. Some of the manual discrepancies could be resolved if the sponsor had access to the CRFs. While the CROs may be imaging the CRFS at this time, it is unusual for sponsors to have access to those CRF images during the course of the study. It does not hurt to ask if they could be made available and, if they are, many questions could be resolved without further checking.

In addition to reviewing data, the sponsor data management liaison must check that AE coding and SAE reconciliation is taking place as called for in the data management plan. It is much better to make sure these procedures are being followed during the course of the study than to wait until the end of the study nears.

The CRO should be expected to send ongoing status reports to the sponsor. These will typically cover:

- CRF pages received
- CRF pages entered/cleaned
- Missing and/or expected CRFs
- Queries sent/outstanding/resolved

Sponsor data managers and/or clinical staff should actually be looking at these reports rather than just filing them away. In particular, action must be taken for missing pages and discrepancies outstanding beyond a reasonable length of time.

Should there be special milestones in the study, such as an interim analysis, targeted data review, or transfer to a data safety monitoring committee, the sponsor's data management liaison must work with the CRO staff both on timelines and on the procedures that will be followed. It must be very clear to both parties and to the statisticians involved what state the data will be in. Will reported or analyzed data be clean, just double-entered, or maybe not even verified? (See Chapter 11 for a further discussion of issues related to interim reports.)

Closing the study

As the time for study lock approaches, the sponsor's data management liaison must be available for questions about whether to query problem data, how to resolve certain queries, and even whether some queries can remain "not resolved" because they affect only nonessential data. This is also a time of heightened data review, especially if review has not taken place during the course of the study. Also, expect a final coding round and final SAE reconciliation at this point; both of these typically need oversight by, or at least input from, the sponsor staff.

The data management plan should already include a description of the procedures that the CRO is following to lock the study. This may be the CRO's procedures or the sponsor's. Both sides should have agreed previously whose final lock form will be used and who must give final permission to lock the database.

After the study has been locked, the sponsor's data management liaison should review all documents in the study file for this project to make sure they are both the most current version and that they are properly signed. (It is not uncommon for documents in CRO studies to be missing appropriate signatures when new versions are created during the course of the study.) The sponsor will also need to secure and possibly load the final data transfer, receive and account for all paper CRFs and query forms, and check images (if any). When the study is finally done, the sponsor's data management group should have sufficient evidence that they oversaw all aspects of the study and can attest to the quality both of the data and the methods used to collect that data.

SOPs for working with CROs

Many companies will have a corporate-level SOP that lays out the bid process and specific requirements for contracting with a CRO. This would typically include the audit requirement mentioned above. If that SOP does not exist, data management can still do the right thing at a department level and push for an audit and develop an appropriate responsibility matrix.

Data management groups that work frequently (or even exclusively) with CROs can also develop a "CRO Manual" to lay out data management's expectations explicitly. The manual would, for example, require a data management plan from the CRO along with all edit check specifications and data management self evident corrections. It would also provide recommended workflows for coding, SAE reconciliation, listing review, and the issuing of manual discrepancies. Besides setting clear expectations for the CRO, a manual such as this provides consistency within data management when different data managers are working on projects with different CROs.

Benefiting from CROs

Getting the work done (and presumably done well) is the main benefit of working with a CRO. The experience the CRO gains from the study and the treatment is extremely valuable and can also be a benefit to the sponsor. When a sponsor provides adequate support staff to answer questions and meet regularly with the CRO, then the experience the CRO is gaining with the study is shared with the sponsor with no additional effort. Small companies, in particular, do themselves a disservice by not staying closely in touch with a CRO during a trial and must overcome their reluctance to provide adequate support staff. After all, the data is all there is to show for the investment in the treatment, and all there is to guide future studies. To benefit from it, the sponsoring company must provide someone to receive the knowledge!

Many data management groups have rules of thumb to help determine the staffing level needed for a CRO study. Some say that one sponsor data manager can handle four or five active CRO projects at a time, fewer if the studies are large and complex. Looking at it the other way, in order to provide time for meetings, review of documents, data review, issuing manual discrepancies, and tracking the project, a sponsor's data management liaison should allocate at least 5 hours per week. (The hours do not add up to 40 in this rule of thumb because some of an employee's hours are taken up by the sponsor and studies will fluctuate in their needs, requiring more time some weeks.) Larger companies generally have the resources to assign someone but may still make the mistake of not allotting enough of the person's time. Small and emerging companies feel that they do not have the staff to provide the internal management, and this may be the biggest mistake they make. There is too much leeway in the conduct of a study and in the interpretation of guidelines to expect a study to be run effectively without ongoing contact. With no one involved with the trial, it is almost guaranteed to be different from other trials being run in house, at other CROs, or even at the same CRO.

Finally, it is worth noting that the opportunity to benefit from a CRO is reduced if the relationship between the CRO and sponsor is adversarial. The sponsor company is entrusting to the CRO important elements of its development program. The success of the CRO is a success for the sponsor. The relationship between the CRO staff and the sponsor staff should not be an "us versus them" relationship but rather a partnership where the combined staffs act as a team. From the sponsor's side, acting as a team means treating the CRO staff with respect, providing information, answering questions in a timely manner, and fulfilling the sponsor task responsibilities using best possible practices. The goal is to deal with the CRO staff as if they were part of the same organization but located elsewhere. From the CRO's side, the staff must care about the details, make note of and track down possible problems, and keep the sponsor informed. In general, the goal at the CRO should be to treat the study as its own.

part three

CDM systems

All data managers work with computer software applications. They may or may not be involved in selecting, implementing, or configuring those systems. In this part of the book, we look at the types of software systems that data managers are likely to encounter and discuss how these systems are put into production. Given the fast pace of software development and the rapid growth (and failure) of electronic data capture vendors, most data managers are likely to be involved, at least peripherally, in vendor selection and validation of new systems.

Discussions of system selection and validation could take up an entire book in their own right. The chapters that follow aim to provide a good overview without going into exhaustive detail or extensive procedures.

chapter sixteen

Clinical data management systems

Except for companies that outsource *all* data management to contract research organizations (CROs) or electronic data capture (EDC) vendors, all data management groups use computer systems to carry out their data management tasks. These are large and specialized applications known as clinical data management (CDM) systems. CDM systems are designed specifically to support clinical data management groups in carrying out tasks over multiple and simultaneous studies.

All of these systems have an underlying database that is used to store the data associated with a clinical trial. The database may be a commercial product, such as Oracle, or a proprietary database built specifically for the application. On top of the database is an application that takes user instructions and applies them to objects in the database. The user gives the instructions via graphical user interface (GUI) screens, checklists, or forms, and only on a limited basis as programming instructions. The system translates the instructions into actions on the tables and other objects defined in the database.

The idea that classical CDM applications support the full range of data management tasks is what differentiates them from EDC systems (discussed in Chapter 17) or other types of data collection tools and applications. At a minimum, CDM systems have the following features to support:

- Database design
- Entry screen creation
- Data entry (though this may be through optical character recognition, single, or double entry)
- Data cleaning through edit checks
- Discrepancy management and query resolution
- Locking of studies
- Extraction of data for reporting and analysis
- Account management and access

Many of them also support:

- Loading of external data including lab data
- Coding against MeDRA and other dictionaries

Where CDM systems come from

Before 21 CFR 11, there were entire conference sessions devoted to the pros and cons of building a custom CDM system versus buying one from a vendor. We do not see these discussions at all any more since systems are generally purchased. The main reason that 21 CFR 11 had such an impact is that meeting the regulations and the recommendations laid out in Food and Drug Administration (FDA) guidance documents requires a professional approach to software development. Most biopharmaceutical and device companies have decided that their area of expertise is *not* in the area of software development but rather in development of new drugs, treatments, and devices. They have decided to leave the development of large systems to vendors.

That is not to say that these companies do not do any software in development. In fact, all of the large and midsize companies that have the resources do add onto the systems they buy. They may extend the base system, integrate the system with other applications, and/or add on specialized reports. Small companies usually have to take the features of the CDM systems as they are out of the box, but they usually do end up creating specialized reports to meet their business needs.

Choosing a CDM system

We look more closely at choosing a vendor product in Chapter 18, but it is worth making one point about vendor products here and that is that they work. When used properly, the systems all collect data that reflect the protocol, store it, and clean it. They also allow for the extraction of that data for analysis. The tasks in the data management process that are easy in a given CDM system and the tasks that are awkward or require more resources do differ from product to product, of course, and that forms the basis for choosing between them.

In the area of database design, in particular, CDM systems do show significant differences. Some are table-based, some are hypernormalized, and others are page based. These underlying concepts and the tools provided for database development have an impact on workflow downstream in the data management process. The database concepts also impact the way CDM systems provide a way of reusing database designs through data dictionaries or standard metadata. The people in data management groups evaluating CDM systems often have a strong inclination toward one structure and approach or the other when it comes to database design and this can have an important impact when selecting a CDM system product.

Using CDM systems successfully

To use CDM systems successfully, data managers have to understand that they all have problems and they will never do everything you want exactly the way you want to do it. However, they do many things just fine.

Because CDM systems come from vendors with professional developers and professional approaches to software development, we expect a high level of quality in the final product. That is, we expect no bugs and we expect a really smooth human interface. That is an unreasonable expectation. Even the best developers supported by high quality software and great quality assurance groups cannot produce a system that has no bugs. Because these people are not data managers, they may not know enough about the real work to implement a feature smoothly. All of the CDM systems on the market have bugs and have problems; they just have different bugs and different problems. The key to success with any system comes from preparing for and dealing with bugs and design flaws when they arise.

We also have to remember that even though CDM systems can be used out of the box, they are installed and configured differently by each company and they have to be validated by the end user. Chapter 19 includes a discussion of configuration, and Chapter 20 discusses system validation in detail. In Chapter 20, in particular, we will see that one purpose of validation is to identify bugs and their work-arounds, but another is to really understand the system in question and adjust business practices and workflow as needed to make the best use of that system.

Sometimes it is necessary to add on a utility or report to make the system work better. Sometimes it is necessary to change the group's approach or lower expectations.

SOPs for CDM systems

The SOPs for CDM systems are those that cover implementation, validation, and change control. These SOPs are often written by the information technology group. In smaller or newer companies, data management may have to create these SOPs themselves.

CDM systems are for more than data entry

Just as data management is more than data entry, CDM systems are more than data collection tools or data entry applications. Even the smaller vendor products will support the key data management tasks for many studies at a time, with lots of data, while being 21 CFR 11 compliant. The larger, more complex (and expensive) systems add on more features for more tasks, greater flexibility, and further options for configuration. They will also be able to handle even larger volumes of data and studies.

chapter seventeen

Electronic data capture systems

Electronic data capture (EDC) systems deliver clinical trial data from the investigation sites to the sponsor through electronic means rather than paper case report forms (CRFs). The site may be entering the information directly into screens without first writing it down on paper, in which case the record is an electronic source record. The site may first record the information on paper and then enter it later. The paper in this case may be normal site source documents or special worksheets provided by the sponsor; the paper is *not* a CRF and is not sent to the sponsor.

In most current EDC systems, the site is online with a central computer and the data is stored only on a central computer. These systems work like, and feel like, the familiar Web sites we visit to shop. As soon as we make a selection and provide payment information, the order is known to the vendor. Some EDC vendors provide systems that also allow sites to work offline. These store the data locally until the site initiates a connection. This approach is much like the one we use with our personal digital assistants that store all kinds of information and synch up with our personal computers when we can make a connection. There are pros and cons to both of these approaches, which we will discuss later in this chapter.

EDC systems are optimized for site activities during a clinical trial and typically feature:

- eCRFs for the entry of data
- Extensive single field and cross-field checks on the data
- Tools to allow sites to review and resolve discrepancies
- Ways for the sponsor to raise manual discrepancies while reviewing data
- True electronic signatures so the investigator can sign for the data
- Record or patient locks on the data
- Tools to assist monitoring

- Reports about patients for the sites and reports for the sponsor about sites
- A portal that provides information about the study to the sites
- A variety of ways to extract the data for review and analysis

What makes EDC systems different?

If EDC systems collect the data and manage discrepancies why are they not considered just another kind of CDM system? The reasons are, in fact, a bit subtle and hinge on certain aspects of performing data management for clinical trials. Some of the key differences between the two kinds of systems are found in:

- The support for multiple trials
- Managing multiple data streams
- How coding is handled
- Where data is stored
- Workflow for study setup

Support for multiple studies

Data management groups run trials (plural); all but the smallest groups run more than one trial at a time and they run many, many trials over just a few years. Clinical data management systems are built specifically to manage multiple trials at the same time. Not only do they support separate storage and security, they also provide features to allow reuse of similar (standard) trial designs or modules, which greatly speeds database setup.

Current EDC systems are very much focused on a trial at a time. EDC studies are built as special applications and tailored to the trial. While they can reuse parts of previous trials, they currently do not provide the full-featured standard data dictionaries that CDM systems provide. Not only does this lead to additional work at study setup but it can lead to a drift in the way that data is collected, which will impact analysis.

Multiple data streams

Large trials often have several streams or sources of data. These include integrated voice response system data, lab data from central labs, laboratory normal values, electrocardiogram readings, and even electronic patient diary data. This data must be cross-checked against the patient data during the conduct of the trial to identify discrepancies or unusual occurrences. EDC systems do not support multiple data streams very well yet.

Even small data management groups store data that is not strictly patient related in their CDM systems. The most common type of nonpatient data is laboratory normals (see Chapter 8). Other important examples include investigator/site information and coding dictionaries. EDC systems are heavily patient-based and not set up for nonpatient data.

Coding

Strong support for the coding process, not just the coding dictionary, is a typical feature of the larger CDM systems. Those systems support robust automatic coding and maintenance of synonyms and provide tools for making manual assignments (see Chapter 9 and Chapter 23 for more on coding). Current EDC systems may only support import of codes after they have been coded externally, if that.

Hosting

Another way that EDC systems are different from classic CDM systems is that the central computer storing the data from the trial is typically *not* the sponsor's computer. EDC applications are most commonly hosted by the system vendor or by some other third party. There are two main reasons for this:

1. There is at this time some uncertainty as to the interpretation of regulations regarding the requirement that a site own or have control of the patient data. Many companies feel that having the data under the total control of the sponsor violates this regulation. Some others feel that a sponsor's own information technology department could be considered an appropriate trusted third party. This discussion will certainly continue for a few more years but for now, most data managers will see hosted applications.

2. EDC applications require a sophisticated technical infrastructure to support high-bandwidth access to the server with 24/7 availability and very high quality security and emergency planning. Many biopharmaceutical companies (rightly) see that they do not have the expertise to provide this kind of environment.

This hosting arrangement means that even though the sponsor has access to the application and the data, a sponsor has to request or perform data extractions and transfers to get copies of the data for aggregate review, coding, and analysis. In this way, the arrangement is more like working with a contract research organization (CRO), but a CRO that supports frequent contact with the data.

Study setup

One more extremely important difference is worth highlighting. In studies conducted on paper with traditional data management systems, once the CRFs have been approved, patient enrollment can begin. Except in the case of fax-in systems, it is the norm to have the database lag considerably behind patient enrollment with no harm done to the project timeline. In fact, as long as the database is ready (not even the edit checks) when the paper arrives in house, many project managers are not even aware how long a database build takes. In addition, edit checks often lag behind the database build. Technical development work is spread out with deadlines based on what paper is expected in house and when.

In EDC systems, *no* patients can be enrolled until the entire application has been built, tested, and approved. The application also includes all of the key patient-based edit checks. This is a significant front loading of the study setup process that project managers must be aware of and account for. Especially in the first few EDC studies a company conducts, a realistic milestone for having the EDC application ready for enrollment is critical and may make or break the project.

The need for data repositories

Because EDC systems do not provide the same level of support for multiple trials, larger companies usually have some kind of data repository. Often this is a classic CDM system. This may be true even if the company runs most or all of its trials using EDC. Smaller companies that use EDC heavily have to create repositories also, but they often turn to SAS to provide storage and cross-study access. They also add in special features such as coding through SAS.

Working with EDC systems

Having data immediately accessible but having it reside on a host computer has a much greater impact than one might expect. An EDC application does not just replace the data entry portion of the data management process and leave the rest unchanged. The workflow for the conduct of the study will change because of the availability of the data and because of its volatility. The data coming in from the sites is very active in the sense that can be entered, changed, reviewed, and monitored nearly all at once. This impacts not only data management but also clinical research associates (CRAs) and biostatisticians.

There is no one way to structure the workflow for CDM systems. All the steps of the data management process still have to be carried out but there is some new flexibility in who does what and when they do it that is not available in a paper trail. The traditional workflow between CRAs, data managers, and biostatistics *must* be reevaluated for an EDC study. Just some of the key questions to answer are:

- Who is responsible for the data set specification associated with the study — data management or biostatisticians, or both?
- Who reviews the data after entry — data management or CRAs?

- Can they review only monitored data or should they look at unmonitored data?
- Assuming the CRAs or equivalent are monitoring the data, what must be done before they can visit a site?
- Does the person reviewing data create manual discrepancies or is that a strictly a data management task?
- Is it necessary to review all discrepancies closed by sites to make sure they corrected the data properly? If yes, who will do this?
- Who communicates with the site — CRAs or data management?
- How and when is the data extracted/transferred — is it the host, data management, or biostatistics? Do they extract daily or at some other interval? Do they extract all data or only monitored data? How about data with outstanding discrepancies?
- Who is responsible for coding and when will it take place? How will discrepancies raised by coding be communicated with the site?
- Sites will need ongoing training. Will CRAs, data managers, or perhaps the hosting company train the sites?
- Who gets to say the data is clean and ready for locking — CRAs, data managers, or biostatisticians?

Each company has to raise the issues before beginning an EDC trail and evaluate what resources are available in each group and what allocation of responsibility will work best for a given study. Perhaps the most important thing to remember is that there is no one right answer. Every company new to EDC, and even those with some experience, should review the workflow at the end of the study (or even during the study, if necessary) to shift responsibilities as necessary to ensure a good working relationship with the sites that leads to data of high quality for analysis.

Main advantages of EDC

Many corporate managers get the wrong impression that having the sites do data entry is the biggest benefit of using EDC. Data entry is rarely a problem for data management and there is usually little, if any, lag in entering data from paper. If the sites are using their normal source documents and transcribing that information into the EDC application, then there is the same problem that paper trials have: they do not do it right away. Once they do enter the data, it has not yet been monitored and so is of mixed value. Therefore, no entry is not the biggest advantage — discrepancy management is.

As we saw in Chapter 7 on managing discrepancies, discrepancy identification and resolution is one of the biggest, most time-consuming, and probably most irritating tasks facing a data management group. Everyone who uses EDC agrees that it greatly reduces the discrepancy management effort by up to 80%, but more realistically perhaps 60%. The reason for the reduction is that edit checks are programmed right into the entry screens so that common errors and missing values are immediately identified to the site. Many EDC systems also include screen level checks that look at data across the fields on an eCRF screen and some can also do more complex checks across screens.

Because of these edit checks, the site is aware of problems right away and is better able to address the issues (and less likely to make the same mistake on the next patient). The job does not go away 100% because some discrepancies are generated by activities that take place after data entry and these must be issued as manual queries. These manual queries come from aggregate checks run over larger datasets, listing reviews, coding, analysis of lab data, and so forth. In addition, many companies feel that they must review all the site resolution to discrepancies to ensure that the resolution was appropriate and acceptable and that any necessary data edits were actually made.

Corporate management and EDC vendors will also say that with EDC you can lock a study in 24 hours. (Twenty-four hours from what, one might ask. Last patient in? That cannot be if monitoring is required!) While a lock in 24 hours is not the experience of most data management groups using EDC, companies *can* reduce the time to study lock significantly. One great improvement is that no traditional database audit (see Chapter 5) is required. There is no CRF to compare against the database looking for transcription errors. The site might have made transcription errors but most of those would have been caught during entry through the edit checks and during monitoring against the source documents. Except for the database audit, all the normal steps to study lock we saw in Chapter 11 must take place and these include resolving all discrepancies, final manual review, coding, and SAE reconciliation. If these are started early enough, the study will lock quickly, but the same is true of paper studies. It is leaving tasks that can generate discrepancies, especially data review, to the end that delays lock in any study, EDC or traditional.

Some problems with EDC

Companies that use EDC systems have enough success that they quickly plan to move more and more to conducting studies using EDC. Most of them, however, will admit that there are problems. Many of those problems concern managing sites, technical issues, or a combination of the two.

Site management with EDC goes beyond the already challenging procedures for paper studies. In addition to all the regulatory compliance requirements and protocol instruction, sites will now need to have electronic signature procedures and forms and ongoing training in the EDC application. They must also be trained in appropriate (21 CFR 11) procedures for using the system and maintaining their accounts. They will also need passwords and password resets (at least until we use biometric identifiers more widely). They will have questions about, or problems with, the application and they may also have specific questions about the design of the study in the EDC application. All EDC studies must be supported by a well-staffed help desk that can provide the technical support and direct callers to someone to answer clinical questions.

Not only must the site staff be trained and supported, site computers must be qualified; that is, the EDC host must verify that the site can actually use the EDC system and make a reliable connection. Some EDC vendors say that a site failure rate is on the order of just a few percent to as high as 20%. While overseas sites are certainly a consideration in the qualification, academic institutions or small investigator offices can also present problems. The sponsor must then decide what to do about the site — provide equipment and resources, or forgo the patients that the site might be able to enroll.

While all software applications have bugs and limitations, sponsors using EDC report that the most significant problems have to do with study maintenance and application software upgrades. Most traditional CDM databases will need at least some minor changes during the conduct of the study. If the protocol changes significantly, those database changes may also be significant. CDM databases are generally set up to handle these changes and companies have processes in place to test and then release them. When changes are needed in an EDC application, it is a more serious undertaking. Any change must be made carefully and it is immediately available to all sites when it is moved into production. If training or notification is needed for the changes, all the sites must be prepared before the change is made available. The logistics are just that much more complicated than for an in-house database change.

Software upgrades are a big deal for traditional data management systems because they require validation, they sometimes require a data migration, and they always require careful planning for down-time when the production data itself is upgraded. When an EDC study runs long enough for there to be an upgrade to the actual EDC system software, the impact is again to all the sites. Sponsors report that despite careful planning, upgrades and associated data migration have sometimes led to (recoverable but annoying) data losses and significant down-time for the sites. These issues will doubtless improve as EDC systems and vendors mature, but the fact that all sites are impacted is something that will always have to be factored in.

Will data management groups disappear?

The answer is no. As we have seen above, the work still needs to be done by someone. Responsibilities will shift and the tasks any data manager will participate in will change when a company begins to use EDC, but there is still a need to have a coordination of data storage and cleaning efforts. Data managers are also very likely to continue to play a role in design of the eCRF, database, and edit checks. They may also play more of a role in coordinating the various data streams from a study to assure quality and timeliness of data from labs, coding groups, IVRS, as well as the EDC host. At many companies, data managers will continue to play their important role as overseers of data quality as they review data listings, run aggregate checks, and perform simple analyses on the datasets.

Some companies that use EDC systems widely have reported that the profile of their data management group changes. They move from having many lower-level staff members for data entry and discrepancy management and fewer senior data managers to exactly the opposite. With EDC, data managers are more involved in study setup and more complex checking and there is less need for junior or less-experienced staff for entry or discrepancy management. They also require more technical expertise than previously. This should be heartening to data managers as it shows a trend to more interesting, senior-level positions being available as we go forward with EDC.

SOPs for EDC

Data management plans (DMP) and the associated study files provide a great way to document differences in workflow or data management processing for EDC trials. The DMP allow a data management group to write down, for all peer groups to review, the required tasks and assess responsibility. However, at some point, SOPs specifically for EDC will be necessary as will revisions to existing SOPs to account for different workflow.

One critical new SOP or revision should cover user acceptance testing for EDC systems. Any group (vendor, host, or sponsor) that builds the EDC application for a study is responsible for validating it. Their process usually requires a user acceptance test (UAT) whereby the company using the system tests the application for that particular study. It is critical that the sponsor perform such a test and go over the study application thoroughly before it is released to the site. If a CRO is conducting the study using an EDC system, the sponsor should require the CRO to perform a UAT. Ultimately, the sponsor is liable for the work performed and the site's goodwill toward a study will focus on the application.

Making EDC successful

To make EDC truly successful, we need to understand how it changes the way a study is conducted. The work is no longer as sequential and well separated between clinical, data management, and biostatistics. The work that the groups are doing overlaps more and there is more room for duplication or, much worse, for a step in the process to be overlooked. In particular, if data management alone is given the task to go implement EDC, the project is likely to fail or at least bring little value. It is when the three groups work together to decide what works, given the company philosophy and available resources, that the project gets off to a good start. Continuing to work together and reevaluating the workflow during the initial studies will have a positive impact on the outcome of the study and on the company's view of EDC.

chapter eighteen

Choosing vendor products

Because software systems have a lifespan shorter than in the past and because new applications are constantly coming on the market, data management groups may find themselves evaluating and choosing between vendor products every three to four years. Evaluating and choosing between vendor products can be a simple process that takes a few weeks or a complex process that can take over a year. The steps are more or less the same, but the time and effort put into the process varies according to:

- The size and complexity of the desired system
- The number of vendor products available
- Company requirements for approval of a system
- Timeline for implementation
- Availability of resources (people)

Even for the same complex system, such as full clinical data management (CDM) packages, one company may commit a year and another a month to the vendor selection period. So it is really the last two points in the list, the timeline and available resources, that ultimately decide how hard or long the process will be. Small companies with shorter timelines and fewer people with time to spare are often forced into a quick decision. Large companies, in contrast, often do take their time, generally because they can, but this is not always a wise choice. At all companies, the process of selecting a product begins by determining what is needed and then proceeds through several selection phases, reducing eligible candidates and increasing the level of detail knowledge obtained at each phase, until a decision is reached.

Defining business needs

The evaluation process starts when a company decides what kind of product it needs. A document describing the needs the product must meet may be a one page bulleted list of tasks that must be supported or a fat document describing the details of each task. This business needs document is not necessarily a requirements document; some of the items listed may be required, others desired, and yet others optional. While most of the items in the business needs document may be required (in that the system must support them in some way), it is worth identifying any needs that are actually desires or nice-to-have options. These can be extremely useful in making the final decision should more than one system meet all the requirements.

When creating the list of business needs, companies should focus on the functionality they want to be supported, not necessarily saying how, to allow for different approaches in different products to be assessed. For example, a business needs document can say that a CDM system must have an audit trail but unless there really is a requirement for it, the document should not specify that the audit trail be implemented through copies of the entire record before the change or through change histories on each individual field. While some business needs will validly be specific as to a required implementation approach, the trick is balancing when to require specific implementations or just specific features.

Note also that the business needs document, or at least parts of it, will eventually become part of the validation package of the application chosen, as it provides material that will allow an assessment of the package's suitability to the desired task.

Initial data gathering

Next, the evaluation team begins to gather a list of candidate vendor products. Friends, contacts at other companies, Web searches, and visits to vendor exhibits during conferences are all good sources of leads for products. The evaluation team or group then gathers some basic information about each these products, which may require making initial contact with the vendor. Because marketing materials are rarely complete enough to rule out (or in) a possible product, the group will likely arrange for short demonstrations.

These early demonstrations should be kept short and to the point. It is usually valuable to let the vendor go through at least a good portion of the canned demo before going into specific questions of interest to the group. This provides the group with a good overview of the product and allows the vendor to point out highlights of the product that the group may not be aware existed. At some point, however, the discussion should turn to desired features. While everyone in the evaluation team should ask questions, someone in the group should be responsible for trying to get a bit of information concerning the business needs. If the group will be seeing more than two or three vendors, a scribe should be taking notes at each demonstration.

There is a good possibility that the group will see something new and interesting, and maybe even exciting, during the demos. Evaluation teams should be open to revising the business needs document to include such features. (The business needs document should not be frozen at this stage of the process and probably not until validation.) Once the business needs document has been reviewed and the demos discussed, the group should be able to narrow down the list of candidate products and vendors.

The next step is usually getting detailed information from the vendors on features and prices through a document often called a request for information (RFI) or request for proposal (RFP). If there are only one or two candidates, then the evaluation team may skip this step and go directly to in-depth demonstrations or pilots.

Requests for information

An RFI or RFP should aim to elicit detailed information from the vendor on how the product meets specific needs or requirements. Because creation of the RFI document, which must be specific to the desired product and summarize the business needs, and the evaluation of the responses both require a large effort, RFIs don't provide an efficient means of gathering general information when there is still a large number of candidates. They work better as tools targeted to a set of candidate products rather than as a method to identify the broad range of possible products.

The vendor response to an RFI also takes time. Some vendors will decline to respond if they have not had previous contact with the company, if the timelines for a response are too tight, or if they feel that their responses will not be given appropriate attention. Companies get a better response from vendors if they have had contact with the vendors first and have notified them well in advance that an RFI is coming. Companies must always make an internal contact person who can provide background information, clarify items in the RFI, and answer administrative questions available to the vendors.

Vendor staff will always, and should, respond to items in the RFI in such a way as to make their product look good. They choose words carefully so that it will not necessarily be clear which business needs are fully and easily supported by the product and which are minimally supported or supported only through custom extensions. While it may seem contradictory, the longer and more detailed the RFI, the harder the vendor responses will be to evaluate.

Evaluating responses

When the responses to the RFIs arrive, the evaluation team combines the new information with the initial assessments from the demos and tries to come to some kind of conclusion. This can be a surprisingly difficult task. Each software package will be strong in some areas and weak in others. It should not even be surprising if all the products under consideration end up being weak in an area that the company considers very important.

Deciding which of two needs, both initially labeled as very important, is going to be very difficult if the products do not support those needs equally well. Some companies have tried complex systems of priorities and weighting. Each requirement in the RFI is given priority, and the product responses are weighted as to how well they meet the requirement. The company then performs calculations or even statistical analyses on the outcomes in an attempt to come up with a clear numeric winner. These numbers help, but the final decision of which product to go with, or to decide not to go with any, will probably come down to a qualitative feel about the product and the vendor rather than a pure score based on features. Many people have found that a gut reaction to vendors based on a demo and an RFI results in the same outcome as a complex numerical analysis.

Extended demos and pilots

If the goal of the vendor and product-evaluation process is to learn as much as possible about whether the product would be successful in the company's environment, then the list of business needs and the evaluation of responses may not be enough. Many companies find that they need some amount of hands-on time with candidate products to really understand if one of them will work. If time is short in the evaluation period, an extended hands-on demo is a good option. If time and resources permit, a full pilot of the product (before purchase) may be possible. Neither demo nor pilot would normally be carried out with more than two candidate products, and frequently these tools are used as a final check only of the most probable choice.

Hands-on demos

A hands-on demo takes place either at the vendor or on site at the company and typically lasts from two to five days depending on the complexity of the system. More of the company staff is able to attend all or part of the session when the demo is on site. On the other hand, it can be hard to corral all the group members of the evaluation team for the entire period and also keep them focused. Visits to the vendor may incur significant travel expenses but they do keep the group more focused. They also provide the group access to more than just one or two of the vendor staff members.

The idea behind the hands-on demo is to see if the product would work in the business environment of the company by using data or examples from actual studies. Another goal is to give the evaluation team a real sense of how the product would be used on a day-to-day basis. The evaluation team comes to the demo with sample data or studies to try out in the candidate system. The vendor can perform the more complex tasks with the evaluation team looking on; the group then takes over the keyboard as much as possible for other tasks. Turning the demonstration into a standard training session usually does *not* meet the goals of the demo.

The success of the hands-on demo will rely on the quality of the people sent by vendor and on the data or examples chosen by the evaluation team. The examples should reasonably represent actual data or structures that would be used in the product after implementation. When appropriate, the evaluation team should provide the vendor staff with the data and examples before the demo so that they can do some preparation or setup to keep the hands-on time focused. Note that for complex systems, it would be impossible to touch on all parts or features of the product in-depth during the demo period so the evaluation team should identify ahead of time which features they most want to see.

Pilots

Larger companies may have the resources to spend more time with the most likely candidate product before they purchase a system, but even smaller companies may take this approach when they suspect that the product might not perform as expected. In both cases, the longer evaluation period, often known as a pilot, is performed on the *one* product the company is most likely to select. (Pilots are more commonly conducted after a product is chosen, in which case the goal is more to identify appropriate use of the product in a particular environment than to see if works.)

In a pilot evaluation, the evaluation team takes one or more typical examples and works through them using the candidate product. Unlike the hands-on demo, the evaluation team will perform most of the work. To do this, the product must be installed on site (or configured on a host) and the staff trained appropriately, which is what makes pilot evaluations expensive. Pilots require significant investment in computer infrastructure and in staff resources.

Pilots are also expensive for the vendor. The vendor will be supporting the company staff with technical support, documentation, training, and general hand-holding. None of this is inexpensive, so vendors usually charge for pilots through a combination of license fees prorated to the term of the pilot plus consulting fees for technical staff. The vendor has an interest in the success of the pilot and will usually provide good support if they feel the evaluation team is proceeding in a reasonable manner.

There will be problems during a pilot. Users will find bugs, become frustrated, and will not be able to do things as well or as smoothly as they imagined or as easily as in their current system. This can generate inappropriate resentment against the candidate product. It is very important to set realistic expectations ahead of time. All team members should be warned about this likelihood and they should realize that other products would have other problems. Setting expectations ahead of time and outlining what must work well will help the team keep the process, and problems, in perspective.

That is not to say that the user experiences should not be taken seriously. An evaluation period at the end of the pilot must allow the users to provide their input in the context of the pilot goals, business needs, and terms of success and failure. Vendors should be given an opportunity to respond to the pilot evaluation by clarifying points, proposing workarounds, and discussing fixes or extensions in problem areas. An important experience to note is that large and even some smaller companies regularly decide *not* to proceed with a product after a pilot despite large investments of time and money.

Additional considerations

Companies have found to their dismay that after they made a decision based on the features of an application, the success or failure of a product was based on nontechnical issues. As much as possible, a product evaluation should include consideration of these nontechnical issues, which are valid regardless of the type of software system or application. They include:

- Size of user community
- Availability of contractors
- Quality of the product
- Stability of the vendor
- Product development plans
- Vendor technical support

The size of the user community can play an important role in the success of a product at a company. If the community is large, the system likely meets many common needs and can get the work done. Current clients may have formed a user group that can be an invaluable source of information about the product, the vendor, and how to apply the product in production. There will be other companies to turn to for specific advice and help, and there also may be some movement between companies of staff experienced with the product. On the negative side, a large user community may also mean that the product is older and perhaps not as technically current as a new product might be. A small community may only mean that the product is new to the market; the product may be innovative and well worth the risk as long as the data management group is aware that they are more on their own.

The availability of outside, independent contractors is often, but not necessarily, related to the number of companies using a product. Outside contractors in data management are used by nearly all firms during times of high workload or to assist in special projects. The need for contractors may be ongoing or just for a short time during implementation of the new system. For new or little-known products, contractors and consultants who are not from the vendor may not be widely available. This may pose no difficulty if the vendor's consulting and contracting staff are available and of high quality.

The purchasing company is ultimately responsible for the quality of the product it chooses to use. All companies should assure themselves, generally through a vendor audit, that the software was produced using good practices and was tested adequately before release. Having said this, it should be noted that audits by different companies of the very same vendor and same product do come up with very different results, so it helps if the auditors have a clear understanding of internal expectations and requirements for the product in question.

Companies are often concerned about the stability of the vendor company. Many software products are built by small, young companies with no history and there is always a risk that the sales of the product will not be enough to support such a vendor. Even large companies fail, are taken over, or decide to give up on a product. There is no way of knowing what will happen to a given vendor even six months down the line from a purchase, but reasonable inquires may provide some assurance or perhaps a warning.

Knowing the product plans for the system in question can make a considerable difference in a company's decision. This is especially true if the timeline for implementation and production use is tight. A company should ask:

- Which version of the software would we receive?
- Is it a stable version or a completely new release?
- On what operating systems, servers, and database applications is it dependent?
- Is there a new version coming up in the near term that will require a migration or a complicated upgrade?

Many companies have delayed purchase and implementation of a product in order to avoid starting off on one version and then having to begin planning for a required upgrade or migration.

Finally, if the product has been on the market for a while, it should be possible to assess the quality of the vendor's technical support. This support should include plans for new releases, bug fixes, and documentation updates, in addition to the usual telephone support and training classes. Many companies consider it essential for the vendor to have technical consultants who are experienced in the industry available during the implementation and validation period.

For new vendors or products, the quality of the support will be harder to assess, and there should be concern that the vendor's staff will be learning about the product at the same rate as the new clients. Yet, more than any of the other business needs, the need for ongoing reliable support must be reasonably met for each and every product by every vendor. After all, following a list of features, are not support and maintenance some of the main reasons for going with a vendor product?

What is missing?

After choosing a product and before moving ahead with a purchase and implementation, companies should spend time to analyze what is missing in the product. This review is sometimes called gap analysis. The evaluation of the product information from the vendor, and the hands-on demonstration would probably have identified any important feature or service that is missing; a pilot certainly would have. Some of the missing features may not be required immediately; others will require changes to business practices. Still others will require special programming, extensions, or support from other applications. Knowing what is *not* there, as well as knowing what is, is critical to successful implementation and can be used in negotiating the contract with the vendor.

Preparing for implementation

As the company prepares to move forward with implementation, the evaluation team can complete and gather the documentation from the evaluation. In particular, the validation process that follows will make use of the business needs document, the results of the vendor audit, and the gap analysis. Also, because a company is responsible for the systems it chooses to use, a short summary of the selection process, along with the key reasons for the final selection, may prove valuable.

chapter nineteen

Implementing new systems

Now that a software application has been chosen for use in clinical data management (CDM), the planning to implement the system begins, that is, putting it into production use. Even the smallest, most contained, of applications cannot be installed and released for use without some forethought and preparation. In some cases, a validation plan by itself will be sufficient. However, any new system that connects (integrates) with other systems and/or requires a migration of existing data would benefit from a separate implementation plan. In this case, the validation plan is just one aspect of the implementation process.

Appendix D contains an example implementation plan that demonstrates both the elements commonly found in such a plan and also the complications in trying to put such a plan together. Because implementation projects frequently have many different kinds of complex tasks in them, each implementation team faces the question of how much detail to include in the implementation plan and how much to spin out into separate plans. One approach (demonstrated in Appendix D) is to use the implementation plan to document the overall tasks, providing details when the task falls directly under the control of the overall implementation project and providing references to external plans for especially complex tasks.

The elements of the plan found in Appendix D are discussed in this chapter, along with the risks to implementation timelines found in each task.

Overview and related plans

The first step in any implementation should be obtaining an overview of what will be involved in the implementation process. The overview should touch on what exactly will be installed and in what order. The "what exactly" must include details of the software application and underlying operating system, network packages, application builders, or database systems required. It also should include all the necessary hardware, involving not only server and client computers but also associated equipment such as scanners and printers that have specific requirements placed on them by the application.

171

The evaluation process for vendor products (see Chapter 18) involves a gap analysis that probably will have identified areas where integration with other systems is necessary to support a smooth workflow. That analysis will also have identified necessary, or desired, extensions to the system. (If the implementation team feels that the integration and extension points are not well defined, they may opt to require a pilot as the first step in implementation.) The overview of the implementation plan should identify whether these integration links or extensions will be developed as part of the implementation for this package or whether they fall under separate projects with their own plans.

The implementation plan may have subplans or closely related plans that must be tracked and scheduled. The most common related plans are the:

- Project plan
- Migration plan
- Pilot plan
- Validation plan

The project plan (usually developed using Microsoft Project® or an equivalent package) lists all of the tasks in detail along with dependencies, delivery dates, resources, and schedule. When migration of legacy data is called for, and is not simple, a separate migration plan would guide the development of the tools, testing, and data verification (see Chapter 24). If a pilot is necessary, the pilot plan focuses on that project's purpose, method, and schedule. The most important of all of the subplans is the validation plan, which lists the steps and documentation needed to support validation of the application (for more details, refer to Chapter 20).

Essential preparation

The preparation needed before implementation of a system can begin involves getting all the necessary pieces in place. This means acquiring all of the hardware and software identified in the overview. It also means installing that hardware and software and configuring the software application being implemented.

One common problem in the preparation phase is underestimating the time needed to acquire and install systems. In the case of hardware, implementation teams may be unaware that there could be a wait time due to vendor lead times for delivery of popular systems. Even if there is no delay expected in shipping, the process of ordering and purchasing hardware within companies has become so complex that it introduces significant lead time. In the case of software, it may be immediately available, but contract negotiations may take quite a while, especially if special conditions, extensions, or future expectations are in discussion.

The biggest risk in this preparation phase is forgetting the configuration task altogether. Most large software systems, and many small systems, allow some variation in the way the product can be used. Each installing company decides how to use it and configures the system appropriately. The configuration may take the form of assigning values to system and user parameters, or it may require a more complex setup, such as:

- Deciding on and setting workflow states
- Developing algorithms (as for autocoders)
- Loading large coding dictionaries
- Providing company specific information (e.g., addresses, protocols, company drugs)

The configuration tasks needed for a given software product are frequently difficult to judge and difficult to perform because new users may not understand a product well enough to know what to configure and how. Implementation teams aware of the potential for problems in configuration can try to plan for it by working closely with the vendor to determine what needs to be done and roughly how long it should take.

Integration and extensions

The overview of the implementation plan in Appendix D demonstrates the integration links and extensions that are considered integral parts of the system. Figure 19.1 lists some examples of integration points and extensions that might apply to a CDM system. An individual section for each integration point or extension allows the implementation team to deal with and track each one separately. While integration points and extensions can be very well defined, they are often hard to schedule. Some of this is due to a need for detailed knowledge of the systems in question, but it is also because of the normal problems of scheduling delivery of software. This is especially true if vendors or outside contractors are responsible for the work.

Possible integration points and/or extensions to a CDM system:

- Adverse event (AE) and drug-coding applications
- Lab data or assay systems
- CRF tracking applications
- External data-checking programs
- Imaging systems
- Protocol project management
- Serious AE systems
- Data warehouse transfers
- Clinical research associate tools and reports

Figure 21.1 For a large CDM system, the integration points link the data to other systems. Extensions to the system fill in support for elements of the data management process not supported by the system.

Delivery of integration links or extensions can cause serious problems with implementation plans when the implementation team expects that the software will be mostly all right as delivered and expects to test, looking mainly for bugs. A common occurrence is for the implementation team to receive the software and find that there has been a major misunderstanding. To avoid this kind of major glitch, implementation teams should arrange for a delivery of an early version of the software integration or extension piece, or even a prototype, early in the development process and perform a quick test to look for general correctness of the application.

Migration of legacy data

When new systems or applications are to replace existing ones, the question arises as to what to do with the data stored in the existing system. Sometimes, the old data (legacy data) can be archived and need not be moved to the new system, but frequently, the legacy data must be moved into the new system. This process is called migration or conversion. (See Chapter 24 for a detailed discussion of the issues around migration.) Because migration is such a complex process, it is usually governed by a separate migration project plan that can have a significant impact on an implementation project.

The biggest question the team must address is when to migrate the data in relation to the system or application going into production. In some cases, the migration has to take place before production because the existing data must be available immediately. Serious adverse event systems and autocoders (using existing dictionaries) often fall into this category. In many other cases, the legacy data is not needed immediately and can be migrated after the system is released for production. Clinical databases often fall into this category.

Both approaches to timing of migration of data have risks. Migration before production may turn up significant problems or necessary changes at the very last moment before production. Dealing with these problems would certainly delay the release date. Migration performed after production work has begun means that those very same problems may turn up after production release, which might have an even more serious impact. Also, later migration or a migration spread out over time means that the old system must be kept running in parallel during that entire period.

Benefiting from pilots

Some pilots are performed as part of a product selection process. These determine whether the system or application would meet the company's needs, identify necessary extensions and integration links, and point out necessary changes to business practices (see Chapter 18). Other pilots take place after a selection has been made as part of the implementation project, in which case the pilot's goals tend to be some combination of:

- Determining how well the entire system works together
- Testing, and/or identifying, new business practices
- Updating standard operating procedures (SOPs)
- Confirming configuration choices
- Identifying (and/or creating) necessary standard objects

Pilots during implementation rarely result in the system being rejected but otherwise share many of the characteristics of pilots during the selection process.

A pilot plan helps both the implementation team and those working on the pilot understand the goal and scope of the effort. The plan also provides the information the implementation team needs to schedule the pilot's place in the overall implementation plan. Besides stating the goals or purpose of the pilot as outlined above, a pilot plan would likely include information on the:

- Data or examples to use
- Staff resources and training plan
- Functions, interfaces, and extensions to exercise
- Expected outputs of the pilot

One very important variable to specify in the pilot plan is whether the requirement is to completely process the data selected for the pilot (e.g., code all the terms if the application is an autocoder or enter and clean all the data if the application is a data management system), to touch on a certain set of features or functions, or to work until an end date.

When resources permit, the data or examples for a pilot usually come from a closed study or from a study that will be conducted in parallel in both the existing system and the new system. Because of lack of resources, many companies choose to use active studies for the pilot, that is, the studies that will be conducted in the pilot contain production data. Great care must be taken in scheduling such a pilot in relation to validation. If the company decides to pilot on production data before validation, steps must be included to demonstrate the validity of the data. For a CDM system, this could include, at a minimum, a 100% audit of clinical study data against case report forms (CRFs). For an autocoder, this might involve a complete recoding after the system has passed validation.

The outputs of the pilot should specifically address the goals. If the goal is to determine how well the system works with its integration points and extensions or to test new business practices, the output may take the form of a report summarizing experiences of the pilot team. If the goal is to evaluate existing SOPs, the output make take the form of a list of existing SOPs, whether they require updates, and what new SOPs are needed. If the goal is to confirm configuration choices, the output can use the starting configuration values and approve them or recommend modifications. When a goal is to identify and create standard objects, a printout of the work completed, plus a summary of what additional work is required, would make a good output.

An evaluation meeting should be part of every pilot. At the meeting, the pilot team and the implementation team should review the outputs of the pilot. They should also record user input and comments on how well the system worked. The implementation team should expect that the evaluation of the pilot experience will result in some changes to the system, whether they are minor or major. Until the pilot evaluation is completed, the schedule for the final phase of the implementation, the move to production, would have to be considered tentative.

Validation

As we see in greater detail in Chapter 20, validation is not just testing prior to production use; it is a process with a series of steps that start even before installation of the software product. The implementation team needs to be sure that a validation plan is started early in the process and approved before the major milestones, such as installation, take place.

Near the end of the validation process, the testing will be completed and someone will write a testing or validation summary. This document will summarize the outcome of the testing and highlight any existing bugs, with workarounds, or any special restrictions placed on the use of the product (e.g., perhaps a particular feature cannot be used). The start of production use cannot begin until this summary has been reviewed and signed and appropriate actions have been taken. However, preparation for production use can begin prior to the end of validation.

Preparation for production

As release for production nears, implementation teams will focus on high-profile tasks of setting up the production environment. However, teams frequently forget to include some preparation tasks that mean the system or application is not actually ready on the day it is released for production, causing much frustration among the users. These additional tasks include:

- Updating and completing SOPs and guidelines
- Setting up user accounts; granting permissions and access
- Scheduling customized training and refresher courses
- Satisfying any user acceptance requirements in the production area
- Identifying which studies or data will use the system first (roll-out plan)

The move to production is a critical period for any system, even small applications. The more people with experience on the system who are available during this critical time, the better. For systems built in house, the developers should be on call. For vendor systems, arrange for special coverage by a consultant or technical support. The implementation team and pilot team can also provide invaluable assistance and hand-holding.

Successful implementation

Most companies are aware of the validation requirements for systems and software applications. They will dutifully create and carry out a validation plan for a new piece of software but the implementation may still fail. That is, the productive production use of the system may be delayed if no one takes a step back from validation and sees how the new (validated) software will fit into the bigger picture of data management in a company and all the little reports and connected systems that data management uses.

chapter twenty

System validation

Despite the fact that the Food and Drug Administration (FDA) has required validation of computer systems used for electronic trial data handling in clinical trials since 1996 (see International Conference on Harmonization [ICH] Good Clinical Practice (GCP) section 5.5.3), there is still confusion as to what validation is and when it is required. There are entire courses, seminars, and books devoted to this topic, as well as FDA guidance documents. Because it is such a large topic, this chapter will only present a very high-level introduction to the concepts of, and approaches to validation. Since most data managers will be involved in validation of vendor products, the focus will be on validating purchased systems rather than validation for systems and large software applications developed in house.

What is validation?

We can find the FDA's definition of validation in its "Glossary of Computerized System and Software Development Terminology." There, validation is defined as: "Establishing documented evidence which provides a high degree of assurance that a specific process will consistently produce a product meeting its predetermined specifications and quality attributes." We can also look at the FDA's guidance on validation, which states that the FDA considers software validation to be: "… confirmation by examination and provision of objective evidence that software specifications conform to user needs and intended uses, and that the particular requirements implemented through software can be consistently fulfilled." These definitions are often paraphrased to summarize the validation process as: the establishment of evidence that a computer system does what it purports to do and will continue to do so in the future. These definitions give us the keys to what is required in performing validation: 1. It is necessary to define what the system purports to do, 2. It is necessary to establish evidence that it is doing that, and 3. It is then necessary to provide support so that it will continue to do that in the future.

179

We can see from these definitions that validation, even of vendor products, is a whole process that involves far more than just testing. In fact, the FDA's guidance document on "General Principles of Software Validation" (section 4.2) states: **"Software testing is a necessary activity. However, in most cases software testing by itself is not sufficient to establish confidence that the software is fit for its intended use."** The bold font is the choice of the FDA; clearly they consider this a very important statement to make! The rest of the guidance provides very practical and specific principles that form the basis of a validation.

The validation process starts at the very beginning of system development or implementation when information is collected on the design and intent of the system. The validation process continues throughout development and implementation as details on how the system is installed and configured are recorded. Before it is released, the system is thoroughly tested to document its working and problems. When it is in production use, information on how the application should be used (manuals, guidelines, standard operating procedures [SOPs]) further helps assure continued quality of the product of the application. Changes at any time effect validation status and trigger a revalidation, in full or in part to show that the system is continuing to work properly. All of these tasks or elements of system validation are guided by and documented through a validation plan.

Validation plans or protocols

A validation plan (sometimes call "validation protocol") guides the entire process. It lists all the steps in the validation process, how to perform each step, and what documentation is required from each step. The word *plan* implies an intended course of action. Plans are best written before the action starts and this is also true of a validation plan. Many companies make the mistake of putting a validation task in a project or implementation plan immediately before releasing the system for production. Validation testing may take place at that point but the creation or opening of the validation plan belongs at the start of the process to identify which documents must be produced along the way.

Good validation plans can be used with all types of software systems and levels of validation. The variations are in the level of detail provided rather than in the requirements themselves. While validation plans typically cover the same elements, the names, organization, and grouping of the various requirements vary from company to company (and consultant to consultant). There will definitely be differences between validation plans for custom systems that involve extensive software development and those for vendor supplied systems.

Appendix E shows an example validation plan outline for a vendor product. The meaning and intent of each section in that outline is described below to provide an idea of what is involved in carrying out a validation.

Introduction and scope

The validation plan begins with a description of the system. The description helps readers (e.g., auditors) understand what kind of system is being validated and the pieces that make up the system. Besides a descriptive summary of what the system is for, the text should include details such as:

- Version of the software application in question
- Names and versions of other underlying or required software packages
- Customizations that were performed
- Server types and operating systems
- Client types and related versions
- Network support

These details are particularly important for larger, vendor supplied systems.

An "Options" section can be used to describe what is and is not included in the installation and validation process. It is often easier to state what is not included than what is. For example, certain major function groups or modules may not be used by a company at all and so will not be included in the validation. Certain integration links or extensions may not be included in the general validation plan if they will be validated separately. The scope also provides a place to state that some elements of the system are assumed to be working properly. For example, in validating an Excel spreadsheet application, Excel is not being validated, just the application built using the package. Similarly, Oracle is rarely validated, but applications in Oracle are.

Assumptions and risks

The assumptions and risk assessment section may be the most important section of the entire document. The FDA is heavily promoting an assessment of how critical the software is and, from that, judging the appropriate level of validation and testing required. Section 4.8 of the FDA guidance on "Principles of Software Validation" states: "The selection of validation activities, tasks, and work items should be commensurate with the complexity of the software design and the risk associated with the use of the software for the specified intended use." In other words, work harder on validating the systems and features that are critical to the integrity of the data and less hard on features that are administrative or those that have built-in checks either through technical means or through process procedures.

Business requirements and functional specification

It is not possible to verify that a system meets its requirements in a known manner without stating what those requirements to be met are. Most validation plans now have two sections; one for business needs or requirements and one for functional specifications. As discussed in Chapter 18 the business needs document or list of requirements may already be available from the vendor selection process.

For vendor supplied systems, it is common to refer to the user manual supplied with the system as the functional specification. The manual serves as a description of how the system is supposed to work. It may also be appropriate to include references to release notes, known bug lists, and other supplementary material provided by the vendor to describe the current state of the software.

Installation

The installation section of a validation plan serves to document how a system is prepared for use.

Planning and documenting the installation procedure has proven to be extremely useful to every company that has done it. Even for the smallest systems, a checklist of what must be done to make the system available can help a company avoid unpleasant lapses, assuming the checklist is written before the installation. Note that the installation is often carried out at least twice: once in the testing area or environment and once in the production area. The checklist or procedure also ensures that the installation is performed the same way both times.

For larger systems that come with a detailed installation procedure or guide, the installer should document what choices were taken or where deviations from the standard installation were made. Those notes provide a reference of those choices for future installations. When independent consultants or vendor technical staff perform the installation, companies should explain to them that an installation checklist and installation notes are required.

Many companies require an installation qualification (IQ) process and some also require an operational qualification (OQ) process. (There are some very interesting comments on IQ/OQ/PQ in the FDA guidance on validation.) The meanings for these terms are not universal, but the intent is to assure that the system is completely and properly in place and it does seem to work. The qualification, installation or operational, usually requires some light level of testing or verification of system output. This can be performed using vendor supplied or custom built test scripts or using system test programs. If the installer encounters any discrepancies or problems, these must be documented. These discrepancies may be as simple as forgetting a step and having to go back, or as serious as a complete inability to install. Very, very few installations take place just once, and these notes on problems will be invaluable at the next installation.

Testing overview

We now recognize that the testing portion of the validation process is only one step of many, but it is frequently the most time- and effort-consuming step of the entire validation. Controlled testing, with expected results compared to actual output, will provide the evidence that shows that the system performs in a known way. For complex systems, the test procedures (test scripts) would be found in one or more separate documents. In that case, the testing section of the validation plan would typically provide a high-level overview of the testing approach and pointers to the other documents (see Chapter 21 for further discussion of testing procedures).

Vendor audit

Since the ultimate responsibility for the validation of a system falls on the user, each company must consider whether or not it believes a vendor has provided a quality product when it chooses to acquire rather than build a system. Most companies, large and small, conduct vendor audits or surveys to help document their decision to rely on the vendor's software verification processes. Ideally the vendor audit would take place before the product decision has been made; more typically, it takes place after the decision but before the system is put into production.

The vendor audit should be performed by an auditor experienced with software development as well as the FDA's guidance documents. This is not a Good Clinical Practice (GCP) audit in the usual sense; this is an audit of the vendor's development practices as viewed from the general software industry practices and from the applicable regulations. The audit may be performed by in-house IS/IT (information systems/information technologies) or regulatory staff. The task may be contracted out to a consultant specializing in such audits. Companies must be prepared with a course of action should there be significant negative findings from the audit.

Security plan

Not all validation plans include information on security approaches for new systems. Some companies cover this under general SOPs; others include it in implementation plans or user guidelines specific to the system. When a validation plan does include a security section, the intent is usually to document how security fits into the picture of assuring that the system will run correctly and to show how security will maintain integrity of the data in the new system as per 21 CFR 11. This is particularly important when the system in question cannot fulfill all the needs of tracking who had what kind of access and when, and the group must implement specific procedures to fill the gaps (see also Chapter 14).

SOPs and guidelines

In recognition of the fact that a system includes not just computers and software but also people and processes, some companies include a section on SOPs and guidelines in their validation plans. The goal of the section is to identify which SOPs or specific guidelines will apply to the process, including which ones need to be updated and reviewed. This is meant to provide evidence that the new system is used appropriately.

Completion criteria

When is the system considered validated? A section on completion criteria including what must be in place before a system is ready for production use is essential to determining if the requirements of the validation have been fulfilled. A final test report and/or validation summary must be part of the completion criteria. Associated with the final report should be an appropriate level of sign-off on the process. Large, important systems should require higher levels of sign-off than small systems used by a limited group of people.

Maintaining validation plans

It is fairly common for a validation plan to be changed after the initial sign-off and after the installation and testing has begun. Sometimes the environment is found to be different at installation. Sometimes there is a change to testing based on new information. There may also be a last-minute change in scope. The validation plan should be updated to reflect these changes and normal document-revision procedures should apply. Be sure to obtain appropriate sign-off for revisions, not just the original version.

Change control and revalidation

Systems change and will require revalidation. Revalidation is the process of repeating all or part of the validation process to provide assurance that the system is still running in a known way after a change has taken place. The scope of revalidation is closely tied to the kind of change made to the system. Change control systems track changes to guide revalidation and to keep systems in a validated state.

In the guidance on validation, the FDA explicitly requires change control procedures. Section 4.7 is entitled, "Software Validation after a Change." That section includes the following statement, "**Whenever software is changed, a validation analysis should be conducted not just for validation of the individual change, but also to determine the extent and impact of that change on the entire software system.**" Again, as in the quote earlier in this chapter, the bold font comes from the FDA. There is no getting around this requirement.

Complete retesting may be called for when a major new version of product is released or when there are changes to the underlying database application or operating system. More limited retesting may be chosen when the changes are bug fixes to specific problems. In a few cases, the change is expected to have no impact, so a decision may be made to simply bring up the system to see if it runs. (An example of this later case would be a change in a network protocol underlying a client server application.) Change control approaches are discussed in more detail in Chapter 22.

What systems to validate

A system can be a complex software application developed in house; it can be a small vendor supplied software package; it can be a small user-written SAS program to clean data; it can also be a data management study application built using a software package. Any of these systems that have an impact on the safety and efficacy of clinical data is subject to validation.

At the time of this writing, nearly all companies validate large and midsized custom systems and all vendor systems with direct application to GCP data. Most are beginning to require validation of all user-written programs large and small, such as SAS programs that are used in analysis. More and more are requiring validation of applications, such as study databases and data entry applications, built using software packages but without programming. This latter class of applications is software development of a sort, since the software packages build applications that directly affect the storage and extraction of the data.

The level of validation, that is, the extent of the effort and resources applied, would not be the same for all systems and applications. The effort for complex custom systems would be very high indeed. The effort for widely used vendor systems would be somewhat less (since there can be some reliance on the vendor materials). The effort for small user-written programs and application-built systems would likely be minimal. However, all validation efforts do need to cover the same points and to provide the same assurance of quality. They must include:

- Requirements and specifications
- A plan to carry out the validation
- Test procedures to provide evidence of proper function
- A summary stating requirements were met
- Change control to provide continued validated functioning

"What!?" companies ask, "Are you saying we need a validation plan for every database we build?" Well, yes actually, but there are short cuts for such things. In the case of a database application built in a validated clinical data management system, the validation requirements can be met as follows:

- An annotated CRF plus requirements for hidden fields acts as the specification
- An SOP on building and testing a study database acts as the validation plan
- The normal entry and data cleaning testing is filed as the evidence
- A "ready-for-production form acts" as the summary of testing
- Change control should be in effect in any case

See Chapter 4 for further discussion of study level validation and Chapter 10 for validation of reports.

It is worth finishing this section with a reminder to apply risk assessment appropriately. It really is not necessary to go through validation for little reports or programs that simply provide information. The developer will, of course, test these programs in the normal way but they need not go through formal validation. Reports, utilities, extensions, and customizations that might have an impact on the data should be validated, but at a level appropriate to the risk they have on the integrity and interpretation of the data.

Requirements and benefits

Validation of computer systems and applications that are used to handle clinical data is required by the FDA. There are no exceptions for old, small, or vendor systems. There are no exceptions based on the size of a company; that is, "We have no resources/staff" is not acceptable.

One or two carefully constructed validation plan outlines can be written to guide the validation process for a wide variety of applications. Small or low-risk systems can have low levels of detail or effort; large or high-risk systems can use the same outline with higher levels of detail and effort and more references to related documents.

Until one has gone through the validation process several times, it is hard to see any value to it beyond meeting FDA requirements. There is, however, considerable value! The whole process of validation helps everyone involved with a software application understand what the system does, how it was built, how it should be run, and what must be done to keep it running. Also, because all software systems have bugs, validation shows where there are flaws and how to work around them. All of this leads to more consistent use of software applications and a higher quality of the data handled by them.

chapter twenty one

Test procedures

As we saw in Chapter 20, one step in the system validation process is testing to provide evidence that the system behaves as it is expected to. For larger systems, such as clinical data management systems, this is a huge job. First, the scripts have to be developed. This can take months even if people are dedicated to the task. Then after the tests are ready, and the validation process has actually started, the scripts have to be run in the test environment. Because this is a critical point in the validation process, all eyes are on the testers and the test outcomes. The pressure is on because everyone is watching the timelines to move the system into production and stress levels rise every time a problem is encountered. From the practical point of view, no matter how much we talk about the validation process, the success and smooth implementation of a software application or system ride on the testing.

This chapter aims to help data management groups get the most out of testing by setting up appropriate test procedures or scripts and carrying them out in such a way as to really provide documented evidence of how the system works. While the approaches discussed here apply most closely to larger system validation efforts, they do also apply to the testing (including user acceptance testing) of other software applications.

Traceability matrix

We cannot even begin to write test scripts until we know what it is that will be tested during this validation and what it is supposed to do when we try it. Good testing practice starts with a traceability matrix. The user requirements and the functional specifications of the product are reconciled with the list of features or options that will not be used, to come up with a list of things that must be tested. This list provides us with the first column of a table or matrix; additional columns indicate where the expected behavior for that feature or function can be found in the specifications. As the scripts are written or laid out, the applicable script and procedure identifiers are added to the matrix. So, for example, if a data management group needs to be able to perform double data entry with third party arbitration, a few rows of the test matrix might look like those found in Figure 21.1.

It is currently a common practice to specifically list 21 CFR 11 requirements in the traceability matrix. That is, companies explicitly add applicable requirements from the 21 CFR 11 regulation to the matrix. For example, they may list "time-stamped automatic audit trail," or "procedures to restrict access to authorized users" and identify the scripts in which those features are tested.

Test script contents

Each script or test procedure has a header. That header repeats information from the traceability matrix to identify what is being tested and what functional specification applies. The header may also include information on the applicable software version, the original writer, and perhaps change information. Scripts also need to identify the prerequisites. This should include what other scripts must be run first, what test data is required, and whether any external files are needed. By reading the header and prerequisites, the tester should know exactly what is needed before the script can be run.

The different ways companies choose to specify the actual steps to follow in the script vary in their level of specificity. Some companies may choose to specify the actions to perform in such detail that someone largely unfamiliar with the systems can still carry them out. Other companies will describe the actions at a much higher level for knowledgeable users. For example, an action at a high level might be described as "Enter the test data for the first 10 pages of the CRF." The same action with more detailed steps might be written as:

- Select the Enter function
- From the Subject menu, select Register
- Select Page 1
- Enter the data as shown and click on SUBMIT

And so on. The level of detail describing the action is dependent not only on the target tester, but also on the level of detail required by the outcome

Feature/ Requirement	Specification	Tested in:
Two-pass Entry	Data Entry Manual, Chapter 2, pages 22–28	Test Script 2, procedures 1 (first pass) and 2 (second pass)
Arbitration	Data Entry Manual, Chapter 3, pages 31–40	Test Script 2, procedure 3

Figure 21.1 Two rows from a traceability matrix covering double data entry for a purchased clinical data management system. (This example assumes that the correct storage and retrieval of the entered data is tested separately.)

of the test. If a company wants to have a pass/fail outcome on each substep of the instruction "enter pages 1–10," then the substeps will have to be listed in detail.

Obviously, the amount of effort needed to create the different levels of test script detail will increase hugely depending on the amount of detail found at each step. Each company should determine what level of knowledge the testers will have and what level of detail for outcome is required and choose appropriately. Note that the level of detail can vary from test procedure to test procedure as seems appropriate to the test.

Each step in the test procedure needs to have an expected outcome described. The expected outcome may be as simple as "the window pops up" or "the patient is enrolled," or as detailed as a list of all the data fields that are expected to be produced by a running autocoding over an adverse event term. In addition to indicating that the step passed or failed, the user will often be asked to generate a report or print something from the screen as evidence that the outcome was as expected. This is valuable evidence that the test was run and the result was as expected. However, it is probably not valuable to ask the users to do a print-screen at each step. Choosing the appropriate points to provide evidence is an art of balancing proof against needlessly slowing the testing down.

Most scripts are designed to be printed. The paper copy acts as the place on which to record results during the actual testing. That means that in addition to a description of the expected results, the scripts must have a place to record actual results. Because space is limited, this usually means only short outcomes, object or file names, subject identifiers, or other short texts will fit. Longer outcomes, such as screen prints, reports, or listings are printed and collected with the script.

The script printout used to record results should also have a place to record a description of what happened if the step outcome is not as expected. Again, because of space limitations, the testers may be asked to indicate that the outcome was not as expected for that step and then to record details of the discrepancy in an incident log associated with that script. These incidents will then be reviewed and researched by a second person (see later).

Purchasing test scripts

Given what a large job it is to create test scripts, many companies try to buy test scripts from the vendor or obtain test scripts from consultants. The Food and Drug Administration does not look favorably on relying on vendor test scripts because they lack independence of review; that is, the vendor has a vested interest in having the validation test scripts pass. Small companies may consider purchasing a set of scripts from the vendor but they then must show that all the scripts have been reviewed and any deemed missing have been created. The same is true for using consultants. While independent consulting companies do provide a more objective level of testing, the purchasing company should review the scripts created or delivered by the consultants to assure themselves that the testing adequately covers the critical functions at a level that provides sufficient evidence of proper working. There is no getting around the fact that the company using the software is ultimately responsible for its validation.

Training for testers

Plan on training the testers in how to test, not just on how to use the system. Testers need to understand that finding problems is a good thing and not a bad thing to be avoided. The goal is to identify all possible issues, within reason, of course, to make sure there are no large problems hiding behind seemingly insignificant discrepancies in expected results.

Train the testers to read the header of the test script first and then review all the steps before carrying them out. Before starting a test script, the tester must make sure that all the prerequisite steps have been met and that all test data and external files are present. The tester should also be sure he or she understands the steps to be carried out and the kinds of output the script requires.

Testers also need to be instructed on how to fill out the test script results and label output documents. Explain to the testers that these are regulated documents. They should always use pen and sign and initial as required. They should use actual dates. Testers should never:

- Use pencil or white-out
- Transcribe their messy original results to a clean copy of the script
- Rerun the script without checking with a reviewer

All printed output from the testing must be labeled with enough information so that it can be linked to the step that was carried out to create it. They may also be instructed to initial and date the printouts. Proper identification also applies to electronic (file) output, but in this case the identification may be through the file name as the user should not modify the actual output file.

All testers should know what to do if there is a discrepancy between the expected outcome of a step and the actual outcome. Training should emphasize that the tester must provide enough information for a reviewer to understand what happened and what steps came right before the incident. Testers need to know that they should not continue after a system error message. Rather, they should stop and contact the responsible reviewer to see if the test, or even all testing, must be halted.

Reviewing results

Most validation testing does not need to be witnessed as it is conducted. That is, a reviewer typically does not need to be looking over the shoulder of the tester to confirm results on the spot. However, the idea of an observer or on-the-spot reviewer may have value at very high-risk points where the outcome would affect all other procedures. This situation tends to come up more during installation and operational testing phases than it does during validation testing.

For validation testing, a reviewer should go through all the scripts and all associated output as soon after the script was run as is feasible. While going through the scripts, the reviewer should read all the user outcomes and make sure they make sense; there is always a possibility that the tester misunderstood the step instructions and went astray without realizing it. The reviewer may also spot cases where the tester reported an outcome that seemed ok at the time but looks suspicious in the context of the results of test completion. This may be a discrepancy that should be added to the incident log for this script.

After reviewing the results and output, the reviewer turns to any discrepancies or incidents associated with the script. Many companies have a separate tracking document or tracking system for these incidents. The reviewer adds the incident (with its identifying information that connects it back to the script) and begins to research the cause. Discrepancies are not necessarily bugs in the system. They may be due to user errors or script errors. They may also be surprising but expected behaviors. Of course a discrepancy may be real bug or flaw in the system.

In addition to determining the cause of the discrepancy, the reviewer determines the appropriate action. For user errors, the script may or may not have to be rerun. For script errors, the script may have to be revised and may, or may not, have to be rerun. For surprising behaviors or bugs, the reviewer may need to be in contact with the vendor. When the incident is a real bug, the resolution would be a bug report and a workaround if any (including training). On occasion, there may be no workaround and an entire feature may have to be declared off limits and business plans appropriately revised. Most rarely, a bug would be so serious as to prevent the system from being used.

Clearly, the reviewer's job is a critical one. A person assigned to the role of reviewer should be one of the people most experienced with the system being tested. That person should also have established a means of contacting the vendor (via hot-line, or email) *before* the testing begins. In some cases, companies may want to arrange special technical support from the vendor for the reviewer during testing.

Test outcome

Testing is hugely useful. If the system is one that is new to the company, testing gives a wider audience a chance to put their training into use and become familiar with the behavior of the software. If the testing is for an upgrade, users may think the testing is a waste of time. This is not true. Testing will provide confirmation that previously reported bugs have actually been fixed (and the workarounds are no longer needed) and will identify any new problems that need new workarounds. Understanding the limits and power of the system will improve the quality of the data stored in it, and reduce frustration of users.

The result of testing will be lost over time if it is not documented. A test summary or a summary of testing as part of the validation summary is not only a good idea but is often considered a required part of validation. This testing summary is not the lengthy incident log that reviewers have been working with; it is a brief summary of the number of problems found and the typical causes. It should highlight actual bugs and focus on any limits to production use that those bugs place on the system. Any special or corrective actions taken should be very clear.

Retaining the test materials

Obviously, the script copies used during testing and all the output and outcomes, along with the incident log and testing summary, must be retained as evidence of the validation. It is also vital to keep the test scripts in their electronic form. All systems will need to be revalidated all or in part when changes such as patches, bug fixes, and upgrades are made to the software product itself or to underlying base software. As we see in Chapter 22, each change will be evaluated to see what level of testing is required. The best kind of testing is regression testing where the original scripts that were previously run are run again, with the results expected to be the same. An essential part of regression testing is having access to the electronic versions of the scripts as well as to previous output.

chapter twenty two

Change control

In Chapter 20, we learned that validation is commonly understood to mean: "The establishment of evidence that a computer system does what it purports to do and will continue to do so in the future." The process of validating a system involves defining what the system purports to do, establishing evidence that it is doing that, and then providing assurance that it will continue to work correctly in the future. Modifying a system may change what it purports to do, which will leave it in a state of having no evidence that it is still doing what it is supposed to do. Change control provides the framework for ongoing documentation of what the system should do and providing evidence that it does do it. The change control process, or change management process, as it is sometimes called, process involves documenting needed changes, implementing the changes, and testing the impact of the change.

Change control, quite simply, is required for validated systems. In the Food and Drug Administration's (FDA's) guidance on "Computerized Systems Used in Clinical Trials," section IX.C deals with change control specifically. The FDA says, "We recommend that the effects of **any changes** to the system be **evaluated** and a decision made regarding whether, and if so, what level of validation activities related to those changes would be appropriate." (Author's emphasis added.) This statement nicely summarizes what is required. In this chapter, we will discuss the requirements in a bit more detail by looking at what falls under change control and exactly what issues should be covered in evaluating the impact of each change.

While change control for large systems is frequently the responsibility of information systems/information technology (IS/IT) groups, at smaller companies data managers may hold responsibility for tracking changes to data management systems. Even at larger companies, data managers should understand the change control system to provide guidance for systems they use on recommended changes and related testing. They may also be responsible for tracking and implementing changes made through data management applications, such as those that set up studies (see also Chapter 4).

193

What requires change control?

Any and all validated software applications or systems require change control. That seems simple enough, but it is important to understand that larger systems and applications are more than a single program, package, or application. Those systems incorporate hardware, computer operating systems, and associated applications such as databases and even compilers. Generally, a change to any of the underlying parts of an application must be viewed as a change to the system itself and be subject to change control.

Validated user applications are also subject to change control, but are often forgotten. Since many database designs for clinical trials built using data management systems are subject to validation (see Chapters 4 and 20), these would also be subject to change control. This may still be a radical idea for many data management groups who will release a study into production and then neglect to record and evaluate changes. Lack of change control frequently leads to inconsistencies in data already collected and stored.

What is a change?

To track a change, we must first consider what defines a change. For software systems, applications, and programs, anything that:

- Introduces new versions of software
- Implements bug fixes in the program source code
- Implements bug fixes in the form of patches
- Affects system or site configuration files or parameters
- Modifies database objects
- Impacts entry screens or other data collection methods

should be considered a change. The first three bullet points cover changes to the system or application software directly and are easy to understand. The last three bullets are often overlooked because they do not change the installed software. They do, however, impact how the system is used and how data is collected and stored. The idea is to apply a change control to a wide variety of modifications with emphasis on anything that might possibly affect the storage, retrieval, or analysis of safety and efficacy data.

In user applications, including study databases, modifications or additions to the structures once the system is in production should be tracked. This would typically include:

- Support for new fields
- Changes to allowed codes for coded items
- Any other modification or removal of a database field including changes in width
- Changes to entry screens of all types

- New, deleted, or otherwise modified programs for calculated items
- New, deleted, or otherwise modified data cleaning rules or programs

It would usually *not* include:

- Addition of new users or changes in permissions (as this is usually recorded elsewhere)
- Any changes made prior to a study being released to production
- New objects created to support a new study

In the case of both changes to system software and changes to user applications, data managers may cry: "But, but, my change won't impact the data!" That may be true, but that is what evaluation of the change is all about. Always record all changes and then evaluate what impact the change will have (it may be none) and assess the necessary testing as described in the next section.

Documenting the change

Change control systems in use today take all sorts of forms. Some are totally on papers, others are simple spreadsheets or databases. Yet others are full-featured, dedicated applications. Whatever method is used to track the proposed changes, the change control procedure describes all proposed changes, assesses the expected impact of each change, and determines the testing appropriate for that change.

Describe or propose the change

In describing the change to be made, include:

- The name of the system(s) or application(s) affected
- A high-level description or summary of the change
- A detailed description of the change and how it is to be implemented

In identifying the system, there may be one entry covering all affected systems or one entry for each system. The high-level description is used to identify the change but not provide all details. In some cases, there may be a list of typical changes to choose from when filling out this information. The detailed description of the change may fit into an allocated space or may require a separate document, in which case the description would point to the file or document. The method of implementing the change is not necessarily the same as how to make the change. For example, if the change involves replacing a value in a configuration file with another, it may be put in place by copying a file to a specified location, running a special configuration program, or by carrying out a series of manual steps. The implementation describes the approach that will be used and will help in determining the impact and testing.

Assess the impact

For each change, a user, programmer, or IS/IT staff member assesses the impact on the system. The key point is to assess the risks to existing data or data management that the change will introduce. In making the assessment of the impact, include information on the:

- Amount of time the production system will be unavailable
- Any required changes to documentation
- What, if any, user training is required
- Whether any standard operating procedure is affected
- All interfaces or reports that are affected
- The level of testing or validation required

Going through the questions of impact assessment may help clear up the question of whether opening a validation plan is warranted. The greater the impact, the higher the risk, the more systems affected, the more likely the need for a full revalidation. For small, localized changes, the change control system may fill the need for documentation and testing, whereas it would not be sufficient for covering the information needed for a more widespread change.

Plan the testing

Testing is essential for each and every change, at an appropriate level. Specific bug fixes can be tested specifically against the conditions that cause the bug and against the normal working. Changes that have wide impact may require light testing across many areas or features. New releases may require complete retesting of the system.

For some changes, defining appropriate testing may be surprisingly difficult because they are meant to fix bugs that only show up under rare or unusual circumstances. In these cases, it may be sufficient to find some way to ensure that the change was properly and completely implemented and installed, and then to confirm that the normal behavior is unaffected. Checking the implementation may include printing the new configuration parameters, displaying the changed source code, or showing that a patch is now recognized by the system via a special version number.

As with the assessment of impact, an assessment of the level of testing may help determine whether or not a validation plan is warranted. If a lot of testing is required across several areas, then a validation plan may be warranted.

Releasing changes

Whenever possible, the implementation and testing of changes should take place on the side so that they do not affect production use. This is not always possible, so testing may have to take place in the production environment. Clearly the system should not be in use at that time, and there must be a way to get back to the original state in the case that testing turns up a problem.

When the testing is complete and all other requirements for documentation, training, review, and so on are met, then the change can be released for production use. The release may involve duplicating the change in the production environment or making the production environment available for use. It is important to record the actual date and time it was released for production and to record who made, and reviewed, the final release.

Problem logs

Some auditors consider problem logs an essential part of change control. A problem log is an ongoing record of problems reported by users. When a user detects a bug or notices a problem or inconsistency in the software, that person reports it to the responsible systems person. That person will research the problem and attempt to identify the cause. This research is an essential part of problem log maintenance. For problems that are:

- Due to user error — the researcher may recommend broader user training.
- Misunderstood system designs — the researcher may explain to the user and perhaps also provide feedback to the developer/vendor that this is not a clean design.
- Rare or not reproducible — the researcher records everything that is known in the hope that the information will help the next time the problem shows up, if ever.
- A true bug — the researcher reports the bug to the developer or vendor and attempts to identify any available workarounds or patches. If the bug is serious, and a patch is available, this may lead to an upgrade.

Considering version control

Change control for software or applications written in house often includes an element of release management. This means that each production version is archived and the differences between versions are understood in detail. (An archive copy is different from a backup in that the archived version will not be overwritten. It provides a permanent record of what was released for production.) Implementing release management or version control can be as simple as keeping a copy of the program or application along with a description of what is in the version on a diskette or in a specified directory. Version control may rely on specialized software.

Software vendors routinely use release or version control programs to track changes and document releases. The more sophisticated version control programs can list differences between versions, identify which bugs were fixed in a new release, and otherwise allow for extensive annotation of each release. These version control programs can be used, not only for actual code or executable versions, but also for related files such as configuration or formatting files. Biopharmaceutical companies that produce large systems or significant numbers of applications might consider using such programs.

The value of change control

Change control is another example of a required process that has immediate values for the groups that implement it. The first immediate benefit of change control is to make people think about a change before making it. Often, they will catch their own problems ahead of time or identify areas of risk. If the policy of "do and review" is in place for changes, the reviewer often picks up on potential problems areas that the proposer did not see. Looking for errors or missing pieces before making a change always improves the chance that the change will be made smoothly and no data (or users) will be adversely affected.

Problem logs can also provide a great deal of value. The record of problems over time, possibly a rather long period of time, helps when technical staff changes. New staff members can quickly find known problems. Good documentation of rare problems builds up over time until a resolution or cause can be identified. Finally, the record of bugs and their associated patch or version numbers is used to create targeted test scripts when those fixes are put into place.

chapter twenty three

Coding dictionaries

Some kinds of data is collected as free text but must eventually be grouped together into like terms for review and analysis. The most common examples of this kind of data is adverse events (AEs), medications, and diagnoses. In all of these cases, the investigator reports a term with little or no guidance on terminology or wording. Yet, to make assessments of the safety of the drug, like terms must be counted or classified together. For example, the AE terms headache, mild headache, and aching head should all be counted as the same kind of event. Similarly, the drugs reported as Tylenol and acetaminophen should be classified as the same drug.

The process of classifying the reported terms by using a large list of possibilities is known as coding. The list of possibilities or standard terms is known as a dictionary or thesaurus. (This book will use the term dictionary.) The part of the coding process that is performed by specialized computer programs is known as autocoding, and the programs themselves are autocoders.

Data management always has responsibility for collecting the terms to code in clinical trials because they arrive with the rest of the patient data. Data management may also have the responsibility for the coding process and dictionary maintenance, or these tasks may fall, all or in part, to a specialized coding group. In the case of AEs, the company's drug safety group may also play a role. Generally, data management takes on more of the coding tasks in smaller companies. In larger companies, more of the responsibility for the coding process and dictionary maintenance goes to specialized groups. Discrepancies do arise during the coding process. These are generally registered and managed by data management staff, who also makes edits to the stored data when the discrepancies are resolved.

In this chapter, we look at dictionaries and the coding process and discuss some of the issues surrounding the maintenance of the dictionaries themselves.

Common coding dictionaries

The various dictionaries or thesauri used in coding have different structures but many similarities. There is usually a term, phrase, or name that identifies

199

the AE, drug, or disease in question and a related code. The code is not always numeric; it may be just another text version of the preferred term. Associated with the reported term and code is a grouping term or a preferred term. In addition to terms and codes, dictionaries generally have auxiliary tables or columns with related information. For example, adverse reaction dictionaries have information on affected body systems. Drug dictionaries may have additional information on key ingredients or manufacturers.

In the past, there were options when choosing dictionaries to categorize AE terms. At this time, companies use only MedDRA (see later). There is more choice of dictionaries for coding medications. Many small companies will start with a medication dictionary or list that they develop on their own that includes those drugs most common in their area of development. As they grow they will later move to one of the more standard drug dictionaries.

Government agencies or designated support groups maintain and distribute the paper and electronic versions of the common dictionaries. Those currently in wide use are:

1. **MedDRA.** Medical Dictionary for Regulatory Activities (MedDRA) is a relatively new international medical terminology that is designed to support the classification of medical information. MedDRA is innovative in that it is an international effort and aims to satisfy the needs of regulatory agencies outside the United States. MedDRA goes beyond simply adverse reactions in that it includes terms that describe diseases; diagnoses; signs; symptoms; therapeutic indications; names and qualitative results of investigations (e.g., laboratory tests, radiological studies); medical and surgical procedures; and medical, social, and family history. It incorporates terms from other older medical dictionaries such as COSTART, WHO-ART, ICD-9-CM, and the Hoechst Adverse Reaction Terminology (HARTS).

   The sophisticated structure of this dictionary supports reported or low level terms that map to single preferred terms. These preferred terms in turn have associations with higher level groups and system organ classes.

2. **ICD-9-CM.** International Classification of Diseases, Ninth Revision, Clinical Modification (ICD-9-CM) is a classification system used for standardizing terms for diseases and sometimes for procedures. This kind of term is collected in areas such as relevant history, concomitant diseases, cause of death, indications, and so on. ICD-9-CM codes are numeric; the code is associated with a preferred term text description of the disease.

3. **WHODRUG.** World Health Organization Drug Reference List (WHODRUG) is a dictionary that enables users to group drugs or compounds typically reported under concomitant or suspect medications. The structure of the dictionary has a wide variety of drug names equivalent to the preferred term. These names include trade

names and nonproprietary (generic) names. The codes for drug names, as opposed to chemical names, relate back to the nonproprietary name for reporting. Additional information associated with the drug name includes the manufacturer's name and whether the drug is single or multiple ingredients.

Using autocoders

Basic versions of autocoder programs take a reported term and look for an exact match in the terms column of a dictionary table. These work well with drug and disease dictionaries where the reported terms tend to have little variation. They do not have a high match rate for AE terms where the variation in the reported terms is high. More sophisticated autocoders do simple text transformations on the reported term in an attempt to improve the likelihood of a match to the dictionary. The transformations may include removal of punctuation or removal of extraneous words (such as "patient complains"). Even the most simple text transformations improve the match rate for AE terms.

To understand how an autocoder works at a given company, we have to understand the details of:

- How the term is collected (as this can impact the coding success)
- The results the autocoder returns when it finds a match
- The support, if any, the autocoder provides when no match is found

Collecting the term

The first part of the coding process involves collecting and storing the reported term, which may be an AE term, a drug name, or a diagnosis. The term is reported on a case report form (CRF) or through an electronic case report form (eCRF) screen and is then transcribed or transferred into the database using the normal data management processes. Because the reported term is generally collected as free text (except in the case of signs and symptoms or expected concomitant medications), data management may find some terms hard to read, misspelled, containing abbreviations or symbols, or longer than will fit in the database fields. Company specific guidelines specify how to handle these events in general and data management should be aware how those guidelines will specifically affect the ability of autocoders to code these terms.

All variations in the reported term will make coding, especially autocoding, more difficult. Therefore, there is great temptation to make modifications to the term that will make it more standard. Those changes that can be clearly specified by guidelines may be allowed. For example, symbols may be left out or replaced with standard text (e.g., ↑with "increased"). Some companies permit correction of obvious misspellings based on a study specific, predefined list. Others companies feel that "obvious" is unclear to begin with and that staff without medical training may make incorrect assumptions. As a compromise, a few companies have a secondary internal field, which does not appear on the CRF, to collect a version of the reported term that is more standard and more likely to code. (Of course, this will only work if the database design and/or the autocoder program can include this field in its attempt to find a code match.)

The specific coding process at a given company determines when, after collecting the term, the autocoder is run. Most frequently, autocoders are run after second entry (or quality review). At that point, the entry process will have caught most of the transcription errors and identified illegible fields. When run after second entry, autocoders typically run over batches of data rather than on single records. At a few companies, autocoding may be performed at entry when a term is entered into the database. This immediate coding is more common in serious adverse event (SAE) systems than in clinical data management (CDM) systems, since it would slow down data entry.

It is worth noting that is it desirable to run coding constantly throughout the course of a study rather than at milestones or infrequent timepoints along the way. Coding problems need to be identified on an ongoing basis, just as other discrepancies are, in order to improve the quality and timeliness of resolutions from the site.

Storing the results

When autocoders successfully find a match, they store the resulting code in the database along with the rest of the patient's data or in the dataset extracted for coding. The result of the match may be nothing more than the code associated with the reported term. Some autocoders, however, can store additional information related to the coding process in other fields. This additional information may include:

- Preferred term
- Information from auxiliary tables
- Coding status

Storing the preferred term as well as the code is not strictly necessary as the dictionary can always provide the connection between code and preferred term. However, some companies feel that storing the preferred term information in the data record gets around problems that might arise if the dictionary were to change in a way that the association between code and preferred term changes, that is, if a new version of the dictionary assigns a different preferred term to the code in question. This way, the patient record shows the coding information as a snapshot at the time the coding was performed.

As noted above, dictionaries have auxiliary information associated with a code and this information is typically stored in additional columns or tables of the dictionary linked by code or preferred term. Examples of auxiliary information include body system for AEs or generic name for drugs. As with preferred terms, these do not really have to be stored with the data, since the code can provide the relationship through the dictionary whenever needed. However, the information provides a snapshot in time and ease of reporting and so may be added to the patient data.

Sophisticated autocoders that support a complex process and more sophisticated algorithms often support a field called something like "coding status." The status value in the field identifies how the term was coded. The values might indicate that the code was:

- Provided automatically by the autocoder
- Assigned by the autocoder but manually overridden
- Manually coded

All of these states are used by the autocoder to determine future processing (e.g., never recode a term manually coded or overridden) and by data management reports to identify what coding assignments may require review. For example, many data management groups require review by the medical monitor of all codes assigned manually.

Failure to code

Autocoders and the groups that use them have several options in what to do when an autocoder fails to find a match. Some groups do nothing and rely on manual assignment of codes to those terms. Other groups store information on the uncoded terms in special holding areas until they are processed. Some groups even provide tools to support the process of making an assignment manually to those uncoded terms.

In autocoders that do nothing, the assignment of reported term to code is usually made manually by entering a code value into the patient's data record. This is efficient, and often fast, when the volume of reported terms is manageable. However, the effort involved in making a decision about the assignment for that term is lost. That is, once the assignment is made, it does not improve autocoder matches in the future. When the same term comes in again for the same patient or some other patient, it must be manually coded again. Losing the association also means that the same term may be coded differently in the future.

Autocoders provide major improvement to the coding process when they store the association of all new, nonmatching terms to codes. A manual assignment is still made but that association is stored, often in a synonyms table. The next time that same term is reported, the autocoder reuses the association thereby reducing the manual coding effort and assuring consistency of coding. Some autocoders maintain this association by storing all the terms exactly as they are reported; others store a transformed version of the text in the synonyms table. The information in these tables has further value; it can be used as an audit trail of all manual assignments, making review easier. Also, reports or analysis periodically run over the associations can look for cases where similar terms that really should be coded to the same code do, and that medically different terms were coded to different codes.

Figure 23.1 and Figure 23.2 show two typical coding processes. Figure 23.1 illustrates the workflow when a company has little reliance on the autocoder. In this case, the autocoder is run but if it fails to find a match, the assignment of codes to terms will take place through a manual step in which the coder reviews the data record and edits the record to provide a code. Figure 23.2 illustrates a workflow that makes more use of an autocoder. In this case, if the autocoder fails to find a match, there is still a manual step to assign a code, but the coder updates the dictionary or associated tables rather than the data record. When the autocoder runs again, these new assignments of terms to codes are picked up and stored in the data records automatically and consistently across records and in all future runs.

The advantage of the second approach is that the assignment of term to code is permanent and will be used whenever that term appears again. In the manual approach, the same term will always require manual coding unless the dictionary is updated.

A coding example with minimal autocoder support:

1. A patient reports an adverse event (AE) of "Headache in front."
2. The autocoder runs but does not find a match.
3. A coder manually associates the reported term with "HEADACHE FRONTAL."
4. The coder updates the patient's data with the code for "HEADACHE FRONTAL."
5. Two months later, the patient reports "Headache in front" again.
6. The autocoder runs but does not find a match.
7. A coder manually associates the reported term with "HEADACHE FRONTAL."
8. The coder updates the record with the code for "HEADACHE FRONTAL."

Figure 23.1 An example of the steps in a coding process when the autocoder provides minimal support and the company does not update dictionary tables when making a manual assignment.

A coding process with more support from the autocoder:

1. A patient reports an adverse event of "Headache in front."
2. The autocoder runs but does not find a match.
3. A coder manually associates the reported term with "HEADACHE FRONTAL."
4. The coder updates the synonyms table and associates "Headache in front" with "HEADACHE FRONTAL, which will automatically update the patient record."
5. Two months later, the patient reports "Headache in front" again.
6. The autocoder finds a match and updates the patient's data.

Figure 23.2 An example of the steps in a coding process where the autocoder makes all updates to the data record and the company updates dictionary tables when making a new assignment of a code to a term.

To aid the (still) manual process of making a code assignment to a new term, some autocoders have tools to present lists of potential matches to the coder. The list may come from a simple wild-card match, a sounds-like algorithm, or some other transformation of the reported text. Aggressive algorithms used to present possible matches to a human coder tend to be more acceptable than when the autocoder uses them to make automatic assignments without human intervention.

Special considerations for AE terms

AE terms tend to present more of a problem in the coding process than medications or diseases. In the interest of collecting the problem as the patient sees it, many investigators report the event in the words of the patient. The result is a term reported in nonmedical terminology, with many variations on wording across patients for the very same event. These more complex and varied terms either greatly reduce the automatic match rate or require a more sophisticated algorithm to keep the rate up.

In reporting the AE, the patient may report a series of symptoms that should actually be split into a series of events. The classic example is "nausea and vomiting," which must be split into "nausea" and "vomiting" to code properly. Some companies permit internal staff to make the split, others require that data management register a discrepancy, which a clinical research associate or investigator must resolve. The current industry trend seems to be to ask the investigator to split the term because each term has other data associated with it, such as "seriousness" and "onset" that might not be the same for the two separate terms.

AEs, especially SAEs, may be collected directly by the safety group and entered into a separate safety system. Those reported terms must also be coded. As noted in Chapter 9, the process of reconciling involves comparing SAEs in safety and those in CDM systems to assure that serious events are present in both systems and match medically. If the data management group and the safety group are using different autocoding algorithms or even slightly different dictionaries, the chances increase that the same reported term will be coded to different codes. If they are compared at a preferred term level, this will even out differences. However, even looking at grouping terms there may be differences that must be ironed out by the medical monitor. In an ideal world, the groups will share the same set of dictionary tables, and the autocoder will be the same, or will at least use the same algorithm for coding in order to minimize this problem, but that ideal case seems to be very rare.

Dictionary maintenance

New releases of the common dictionaries appear very frequently. New versions of MedDRA, for example, are released twice a year — a full release in March and a maintenance release in September. Maintaining the dictionaries is a challenging task, not because of technical issues, but because of the impact that changes have. Release notes for new versions must be carefully studied and the impact of the changes understood before the new version is put into place. For example, sometimes an existing term appears in a new dictionary version and is associated with a new code. In this case, data management and safety groups must consider what to do if that term in existing studies has been coded to the old code. Changing the assignment in existing data and locked studies might have impact on SAE reports to the Food and Drug Administration, other integrated safety summaries, New Drug Applications (NDAs), and other analyses.

Every company should have maintenance and upgrade plans in place. One plan is a technical plan for the loading of the data and the verification that it was loaded properly. (This is not a validation plan because typically no software is being installed; only data is being loaded. Data loading for dictionaries must be verified.) A second plan deals with what to do with existing clinical study data. Presumably locked studies are not unlocked for recoding, but their terms may be recoded on the side for summary reports. Open studies may or may not be switched to the new dictionary as that implies recoding and this can impact not only outstanding queries, but also any reports and interim analyses that have already taken place.

Another challenge of dictionary maintenance is managing the impact of the new version on company specific modifications or additions. If a company has added terms directly to the dictionary tables, these terms could be overwritten by a new release, or newly released terms may duplicate terms added by the company. If reported terms that are manually coded were stored in separate synonym tables, these now may code automatically in the released dictionary or there may be a new, more appropriate code in the new version than existed in previous versions of a dictionary. These cases all require evaluation of all synonyms in use. To allow for the most flexibility in support dictionary versions, data management groups should try to configure their dictionary tables and autocoders to support more than one version of a dictionary at any time.

A few more points regarding dictionary management:

- All past dictionary tables should be maintained as archive data essential to the interpretation of previous studies.
- Update access to all dictionary tables should be restricted to those staff members trained in appropriate processes and procedures.
- The dictionaries being used, along with their versions, should be recorded (and the information kept current) in the data management plan for each study (see Chapter 1).

Quality assurance and quality control

Coding assignments provide an important piece of safety data, whether the term is an AE term, drug, or disease. Quality assurance and quality control for the coding process has two different targets: the autocoder and the manual assignments.

Because the autocoder program in effect creates data (the code), it must be held to the highest level of quality development, testing, and validation. Be aware that test data is rarely enough to turn up problems with the autocoder; it is only the variations in, and volume of, real data that exercise the program to the fullest. Therefore, even after putting a new autocoder into production use, companies may choose to review all autocoded assignments for a period of time or on an ongoing basis to assure correct working and quality.

For manual assignments, periodic review of assignments can prevent and detect coding consistency problems. In simple systems, the review may be performed visually as quality control. In systems where new coding assignments are stored, a variety of reports or analysis can help pinpoint areas where similar terms have been coded differently and like terms have been assigned inappropriate codes. Clearly, a process must be in place should an inappropriate assignment be found, keeping in mind that a change in coding assignment may impact previously coded data or data coded in other ongoing projects.

Effective coding

The coding process is most effective when it integrates data management systems, practices, autocoders, data managers, and coding experts. Good data management systems and practices will collect AE terms accurately and will identify many problem terms early. Autocoders run routinely as part of the data handling will also identify problems and discrepancies early. By giving coding experts access to the output of autocoder runs throughout the study (rather than at the critical point near the end), they will have more time to devote to resolving problems and reviewing difficult decisions.

A basic autocoder should be considered a requirement by every company. The more steps of the coding process the autocoder can support, the more effective the process will be. One of the most important features to improve effectiveness is the ability to store the association of new, nonmatching terms to the appropriate codes as synonyms. This increases match rates over time and also helps ensure coding consistency. For highly varied AE terms, an autocoder may have to support complex algorithms to increase the match rate or to make the manual assignment process more effective.

chapter twenty four

Migrating and archiving data

Migrating is the process of moving existing data into a new system. The new system in question may be an entirely new application, or it may simply be a significant version upgrade to a system currently in production. Whenever data is migrated, companies should be prepared to provide proof that the migration did not adversely affect existing data in any way (through deletion, addition, or modification). This verification of the data may be very simple in the case of a version upgrade where the structures underlying the application (e.g., data management system) remain largely the same. The verification, and in fact the whole process of migration, is much harder when moving data to a new system where the data being migrated is transferred to new structures and possibly even transformed somewhat in the process.

Because the process to migrate data to a totally new system may be complex and requires a high level of effort, it is not always worth going through. It may be possible to maintain the old system for a while, keeping the data separate from any new systems, but at some point the old system will have to be retired. At that point, should it be necessary, some or all of the data can be archived in a format that will permit access to both the data and study information (metadata) in the future.

This chapter discusses the more simple migrations, which most data management groups are likely to face, and will also touch on some of the more complex migrations which, though less frequent, do come up. Because the technical aspects of archiving data is quite complex, we only discuss the most basic considerations and issues around archiving in this chapter.

Simple migrations within systems

It is not unusual for a software application upgrade to require a migration of data. That is, the upgrade procedures require that the data be physically copied and moved to another location. A common example comes up when a clinical data management (CDM) system that uses Oracle. Should a new version require a new major release of Oracle, then the upgrade may require a database export and import. An export is a copy. Whenever a copy of data is made, the group performing the copy should be able to show proof that the copy is complete and accurate.

For a simple migration, tools or simple utilities should be able to provide this verification. One tool should show that all of the underlying structures (e.g., number of rows, columns, and tables in a database base) were copied. This result shows that all of the data has been copied, but it leaves open the question of whether any individual data points have been modified. This is at least as important as showing that all the data had been included in the copy. A second tool or approach is needed to provide that verification.

One common approach to providing the second piece of evidence that no data points have changed is to use programs to compare the original data to the final data, value by value. For example, SAS programs that extract data can extract from both locations and compare the results. While the data volume would be high, the actual human intervention necessary to do the comparison would be small. Another option is to use widely available text-compare utilities to compare data extracted before and after the move into similarly formatted text files. It should be cautioned that whatever application or utility is used, that application should have been validated or otherwise verified in its own right; otherwise the result of the comparison may be called into question.

If a data point-by-data point comparison is not viable, some reports that summarize the characteristics of the data may be a reasonable alternative. For example, descriptive statistics on key fields should produce the same result before and after the migration. If you had 346 females in a study prior to the migration, there really should be 346 females in that study after the migration. Programming the statistics to run on each study may be a significant task in itself and often lead back to: "Let's just do the 100% comparison."

Because even simple upgrades can adversely affect data values, every validation plan should include an assessment of risk to determine what level of data verification is appropriate. Once the utilities have been identified and are in place, the actual comparison is likely to be relatively low effort, some level of data verification could be included in every upgrade whether or not an explicit copy is required.

Why migrate between systems?

When migration to a new system looks like it will be complex and require a high level of effort, keeping an old system going for a while seems very appealing. Unfortunately, even simple maintenance and upkeep on older computers and related software packages becomes a problem after just one to two years. For example, should a disk drive fail, getting a suitable replacement for a computer even four years old may be difficult. More importantly, the internal expertise and knowledge of the old application begins to decline even faster, making it hard to maintain and even difficult to access. At some point, it will become necessary to retire the old system. For some applications, it is possible to close out work in the system before that point and archive all the data. In others, it will be necessary to move some or all of the data to the new system before it is no longer accessible.

Consider the case of a new CDM system. When the new system is ready for production use, data management can open new studies in the new system. Clinical studies due to close shortly will likely be locked in the old system. Many of those closed studies could be archived. Migration becomes an issue for long-term studies spanning many years or for closed studies that are part of a critical project and must remain highly accessible. Another classic example, perhaps outside the normal data management area of responsibility, is an SAE management and reporting system. Companies usually require that all existing SAE data be migrated into the new system to assure complete reporting and to allow trend analysis.

Complex migrations

When a migration is not a simple migration, there are usually some options available with different levels of effort required. The least problematic approach simply meets the requirements of the new system but otherwise leaves the structures of the old system unchanged. That is, data groupings, variable names, data types, codelist associations, and other data attributes are left unchanged. Data transformations are performed only when there is an unavoidable conflict between the requirements of the new system and the data in the old (if, for example, patient identifiers must be texts in the new system but were numeric in the old). This method is often a good choice when migrating data between CDM systems. Even if new data structure standards are being put in place in the new system, it is often not necessary (and may be undesirable) to change the structure of existing studies to meet the new standards.

The most difficult kinds of migration are those from two systems with fixed data structures, such as in SAE packages where most of the data structures are determined by the application, and there is little room for variability. When the data structures are determined by the applications, mapping of the fields from one system to the other usually uncovers the need for many transformations of the data. For example, numeric data in the legacy system may be text data in the new; date formats may be different, and codes will frequently differ. Unfortunately, these very complex migrations frequently turn out to be the ones where all the data must be migrated, and it all must be migrated before production use.

Any system that has been in production for a few years and has significant amounts of data stored in it also has significant problems stored in it. There are mapping problems such as those described above and there are also data problems. Data problems are those that arise because the values in a particular data structure, such as a field or column, are not internally consistent. Data problems, in particular, are made worse when the old system already has legacy data in it from some previous system. An example of a data problem is the case of field that was not coded in the past but now is. Old data will contain all kinds of values that may no longer be acceptable.

Mapping problems are really more like challenges in that they are systematic and logical and can usually be addressed or solved through programs run right before or during the migration process. Data problems are much harder to deal with because they deal with subsets of the data that cannot always be clearly specified. In some cases, data problems can be dealt with in the old system prior to migration (through deletion of test data or correction of truly erroneous data). Sometimes the problem data cannot be migrated. In this case, some migrations deal with the data by creating electronic files of records that could not be migrated. Another option is hand-entering those those records.

Migration by hand

The more complex the migration and the more complex the data problems, the more complex the tools needed to migrate those data. Complex programs require time for development and validation by sophisticated and experienced programers. When the job to migrate through tools and programs becomes too big or too expensive, companies should consider migrating by hand, that is, by re-entering the data. Even with large volumes of data, experienced data entry staff may be able to re-enter the data more efficiently than through software utilities. Double entry, in particular, has a low error rate and even 100% verification can be reasonably cost-efficient when carried out by administrative staff.

This migration by hand should be an approach of last resort. Information about the origin of the records (who originally entered them and when) is lost, as is any original audit trail. To mitigate this problem, the original data should be archived.

Migrating audit trails

For systems that have audit trails, the question arises as to whether the audit trail should be migrated along with the data. Yes, it should be. The Food and Drug Administration (FDA) rule on electronic signatures and electronic records requires that the audit trail be accessible for the life of the data. However, this can prove difficult, if not impossible, because audit trails of some older systems are not in a structured form that would allow access and migration. Even accessible audit trail structures may contain less, or more, information than the new system requires.

The migration team should review the audit trail structure and migrate it if the systems are compatible. If they are not, companies should consider putting the audit trail in some other archive format that is perhaps not as accessible as the data in the main application, but could be reviewed if necessary during an audit of the data. This may mean putting it on the same platform or moving only key pieces of data. It is even better to move the audit trail to a different but accessible platform or application (even text files) than to lose the information entirely.

Archiving data

Until fairly recently, companies tried to migrate all existing data through to new systems at every upgrade or implementation of a new application. At some point, this process becomes unwieldy because of the volume of studies and the lack of understanding of the old study structures. When bringing along all studies has low value, a decision is made to archive the data. As the archive structure is designed, the first question that arises is whether the data will need to be readily accessible on short notice or whether it is permissible to require some level of effort to resurrect it. The second question is what should be included in the archive.

Level of archive access

Studies that are several years old but still part of an active product line should probably be available without much effort. For these studies, questions often arise as to AEs or SAEs and these questions may require a review of the study data. There may also be new questions about efficacy, impact on other safety variables, or groupings of patients, brought up by new studies that warrant a look back at older studies. While the data for all submissions will be available in SAS form, there may be good reasons to go back to the original data as it was entered.

The easiest way to make sure data is available is to archive the data to the same platform that the new application is on. For example, if the new system is built on top of Oracle, consider archiving the old studies in a compatible version of Oracle exactly as they were when they were locked. This platform provides ready access through standard interfaces and query tools even if the data cannot be viewed through the new application or system. The archived data is kept separate from production data and under tight security so that anyone who needs to can point to it and read it but no one can make changes. (It should be noted that data for old studies or studies in product lines that have been discontinued, need only be, and should only be, saved for the appropriate record retention period. That period should be spelled out explicitly in company policy and should conform to FDA regulations. Electronic data should be covered just as paper records are.)

When data for studies that are older, or for discontinued lines, still needs to be retained but do not need to be readily accessible, other formats for data archival can be considered. XML, PDF, and SGML are all currently being discussed as ways of archiving data. These and other options for long-term storage are open to consideration. As the FDA says in its guidance for 21 CFR 11 section C.5, "As long as predicate rule requirements are fully satisfied and the content and meaning of the records are preserved and archived, you can delete the electronic version of the records" (by which they mean the original versions of the records).

What to archive

Just archiving the data is usually not enough; if that were the case, saving the SAS extract of the data would satisfy everyone. As we saw in the migration discussion, the audit trail should be retained for as long as the records are (see 21 CFR 11 section 11.10). So the audit trail, at a minimum, must be brought along into the archive. General industry consensus seems to be that as much information as possible about the design and conduct of the study should be brought along as well. This would include database design, coding dictionaries, coding algorithms, derived/calculated values, and cleaning rules. For some systems, this information will be in a proprietary design and cannot be moved electronically. In this case, paper or PDF versions of the information should be obtained before the old system is retired. In other cases, this study information will be available electronically (e.g., in Oracle) and can be archived along with or parallel to the data if care is taken.

Migration and archive plans

Like every other major undertaking we have looked at so far, every migration or archive effort needs a plan. The plan should clearly document the approach being taken for all data and list all of the risks involved. In particular, the plan should specify all points at which verification that the data is true copies will be provided and what methods will be used to provide that verification. For archiving data, the plan should explicitly list all the components of the original system that will be included in the archive and the formats being used for their storage.

Future directions

The whole area of archiving is bound to mature over the next couple of years as companies try out various methods and improve upon standard format models. The FDA issued a guidance document in July 2002 on the maintenance of electronic records, which was withdrawn when the 21 CFR 11 scope and application was re-evaluated. Presumably, the agency will issue new guidance on this topic within the next couple of years. In the meantime, every company will have to make its best effort, archiving as much as possible in as simple a format as possible, and documenting all decisions and approaches for future reference.

appendix A

Data management plan outline

The outline for a data management plan shown here is just one example of the structure such a plan might take. The section headings that appear here come from a combination of actual plans used by different data management groups. The main headings identify the task to be described or the information to be provided. The subpoints provide a bit more detail on the kinds of information that might be included if appropriate. The subsections also list some of the documents that might be created or collected to fulfill requirements.

This basic outline can be easily adapted to studies carried out by a contract research organization (CRO) and studies that used electronic data capture (EDC) rather than paper case report forms (CRFs).

As noted in Chapter 1, the level of detail provided by a given group for a given study in such a data management plan could legitimately vary from little to lengthy. In particular, no information is needed when a task is fully described by standard operating procedures (SOPs) or guidelines. So, for example, if the process for reconciling serious adverse events (SAEs) is fully described the company SOP numbered DM-114, then the text under that bullet point would be something as simple as "As per DM-114. No study specific instructions."

Description

1. Protocol title and study number
2. Reference to protocol document

215

Responsibilities/scope of work

1. Lead data manager
2. CRO contact information
3. Other relevant responsibilities (e.g., coding)

CRF design

1. Who is responsible for design
2. Who needs to sign-off and when
3. How revisions are made, approved, and filed

Study setup

1. Who will design and build the study
2. Computer system to be used (hardware and software)
3. Database design output: annotated CRF, printouts of database structures
4. Entry screen design output: printouts of entry screens
5. File loading outputs: specification, printout of code or configuration
6. Other systems to be configured (e.g., imaging systems, CRF tracking systems)

CRF flow and tracking

1. Study specific handling, if any, for this study

Entering data

1. Study specific entry guidelines — output: data entry guideline document

Cleaning data

1. Edit check specifications (data validation plan) — output: specification document
2. Data management self evident corrections (SECs) — output: approved SECs
3. Study specific discrepancy (query) handling guidelines — output: handling document
4. Query flow and tracking including process for editing data

Lab data

1. Normal range handling
2. Process steps to follow if loading lab data — output: log of loads

SAE reconciliation

1. Process, including discrepancy handling
2. Frequency — output: reconciliation sheets

Coding reported terms

1. All dictionaries and specific versions being used (medications and AEs)
2. Autocoding process and relevant algorithms
3. Workflow for uncoded terms; sign-off required — output: approval
4. Coding conventions specific to this protocol or drug

Other data loading or data source

1. Source of data (e.g., integrated voice response (IVR) data, patient diaries)
2. Frequency of load and format — output: load file specification
3. Process steps — output: log of loads

Reports

1. List of standard reports (e.g., missing pages, outstanding discrepancies)
2. Frequency of reports

Transfers or extractions

1. List of transfers expected or frequency of transfers, if any
2. Process for transfers — output: log of transfers

Interim locks

1. When, if any
2. Process that will be followed at that time
3. Output: what documents are to be filed

Closing the study

1. Study-close checklist — output: signed checklist
2. Database audit plan — output: audit listings and summary
3. Approval process needed to lock — output: signatures for locking

Security

1. Access to application by users — output: access log
2. Signatures — output: signature of users
3. Special security for transfers, if any

appendix B

Typical data management standard operating procedures

The list of Standard Operating Procedures (SOPs) was created from combing through several references to, and sources of, lists of required SOPs. The list is a superset of the topics from those references and sources. It is meant to be a comprehensive list of topics to be covered by a standard procedure. Note that:

- Not all of these SOPs are of the same priority.
- Some of the topics could be combined into a single procedure document.
- Some of the topics might be addressed by corporate SOPs or policies.

1. Data Handling Plan/Data Management Plan
2. CRF Design
3. CRF Flow
4. Database Setup
5. System Validation (and Change Control)
6. Study-Level Validation (and Change Control)
7. Data Validation Programming (Edit Checks)
8. Tracking CRFs
9. Data Entry (and Editing)
10. Coding (AEs and Meds)
11. Query Flow and Handling
12. Handling Lab Normal Ranges
13. SAE Reconciliation
14. Data Audit
15. Database Lock/Unlock

16. Document Management/Study Binder
17. Security of Systems and Data
18. Training
19. Transfer/Extraction of Data
20. Loading Data (from other sources)
21. CRO Management
22. Archive of Study Data

appendix C

CRO–sponsor responsibility matrix

The following table is an example of a responsibility matrix to be used in setting up a contract with a CRO. Most of the key data management tasks are listed; some of them are broken down in detail. Note that this matrix should indicate not only who performs the work but also who is responsible for review (as shown in the first line for case report form [CRF] development). It is also possible that the sponsor and CRO both do some of the work. The matrix should be customized for each study and sponsor/CRO combination as needed to clearly identify the work that is to be done.

Data Management		
Task Description	**Sponsor**	**CRO**
Develop the CRF	X	Review
Print and distribute the CRF		
Write and maintain data management plan		
Specify edit checks (manual and electronic)		
Database creation • Write specifications • Design • Testing		
Programming and validation of edit check programs		
Query management and resolution		
CRF tracking		
Weekly reports • Missing/expected pages • Discrepancy counts including time outstanding		
CRF imaging		
Data entry		
Listing reviews		
Lab data • Receive lab data • Manage lab normals • Check lab data (specify specific checks)		
Database audit • Frequency • Special milestones • Final audit		
Data transfers (how many, what format)		
Coding (specify dictionary and version) • AEs • Medications		
SAE reconciliation		
Approve study lock		

appendix D

Implementation plan outline

An example of an implementation plan outline is shown below. This outline, like that for any implementation plan, is built on some assumptions or knowledge about the particular implementation in question. In this case, we are assuming a single software application is the focus of the implementation. The order of the elements in this example reflects the knowledge that:

- The development of integration links to other applications and extensions will take place under separate project plans and they will be installed prior to a pilot and/or validation.
- A pilot will be conducted and is intended to provide information on how the system works with all of the configuration and customization already in place. It will not be on production data and so can take place before validation.
- The migration element of the plan assumes that there *is* legacy data to move into the new system and starts with a task to determine when that migration will take place: before or after production use begins.
- The validation testing of the entire system before production use will include cases to test the working of all the pieces, including integration links and extensions.

1. Overview/Introduction
   1.1. System Description
   1.2. Goals and Scope
   1.3. Integration Points
   1.4. Extensions to the System

2. Related Plans
   2.1. Project Plan
   2.2. Pilot Plan

    2.3. Validation Plan
    2.4. Migration Plan

3. Preparation
    3.1. Acquire and Install Hardware
    3.2. Acquire and Install Software
    3.3. Configure the Application
    3.4. Initial Training

4. Integration (for each integration point)
    4.1. Initial Install/Implement
    4.2. Quick Test
    4.3. Final Install/implement
    4.4. System Test

5. Extensions (for each extension)
    5.1. Initial Install/Implement
    5.2. Quick Test
    5.3. Final Install/implement
    5.4. System Test

6. Migration of Legacy Data
    6.1. When Migration Will Take Place
    6.2. Separate Migration Project Plan

7. Conducting the Pilot
    7.1. Select Pilot Data or Studies
    7.2. Conduct Pilot According to Plan
    7.3. Incorporate Feedback from Pilot

8. Validation
    8.1. Conduct Validation According to Plan
    8.2. State Requirements for Moving to Production

9. Move to Production
    9.1. Complete SOPS and Guidelines
    9.2. Create Production Environment
    9.3. Set Up Security and Access
    9.4. User Acceptance Testing (if any)
    9.5. Training Users

10. Complete Documentation Packets

appendix E

Validation plan outline

This example outline for a validation plan applies to a vendor supplied software application. It includes elements common to most validation plans but the actual names, organization, and grouping of the various requirements would vary from company to company. This outline shows mostly high-level headings; the description of what might be included under each heading can be found in detail in Chapter 20.

1. Introduction and Scope
   1.1. System Description
        Software
        Hardware
   1.2. Options
   1.3. Project Plan/Timeline
2. Assumptions and Risk Assessment
3. Business Requirements
4. Functional Specification
5. Installation/Implementation
   5.1. Installation Procedure
   5.2. Installation/Implementation Notes
   5.3. Installation Qualification
6. Testing Overview
7. Vendor Audit
8. Security Plan
9. SOPs and Guidelines
10. Completion Criteria
11. Revision History

appendix F

CDISC and HIPAA

New data managers and others concerned about proper data management often ask about CDISC and HIPAA and how they impact data collection. CDISC is a standards format and HIPAA is a privacy rule. This appendix provides a very brief explanation of each as well as links for more detailed information.

CDISC

CDISC stands for the Clinical Data Interchange Standards Consortium. The mission of this independent group is to develop and support global, platform independent data standards that enable information system interoperability or interchange in medical research. Its goal is to develop standard models that still permit flexibility in research.

The group has done most of its work in the submissions data model (SDM). This model refers to standard metadata being developed to support regulatory submissions. The tables of patient data that are submitted with a new drug or device application are submitted using the SDM.

CDISC is also working on an operational data model (ODM) for the interchange and archive of data collected in clinical trials through a variety of sources. This would include not only the data but also the audit trail and metadata (structural and/or administrative data). The important point at this time is that the model is for writing and reading of files for interchange; it is not meant to replace standard clinical data management systems (CDM). However, electronic data capture systems may write ODM compatible files and those files may be read into the CDM system through an ODM reader utility. CDISC also has a lab format for the exchange of lab data that could be read into a CDM system or other data warehouse.

At the time of this writing, CDISC standards appear to have an impact mostly on programmers and statisticians that are considering the SDM. Larger pharmaceutical companies are also experimenting with using ODM in data management and some vendors of CDM systems have demonstrated examples of studies set up to conform with the ODM. For the most part,

227

data managers and builders of data management applications, except in the companies in the forefront of implementation, currently do not have to work much with CDISC standards.

More companies will begin to work with CDISC as more read and write tools are available from vendors. At that point, the impact on a typical data manager will become clearer. Data management groups would be wise to stay current with CDISC. The group has speakers that present sessions at many conferences and also has workshops on the standards. More information can be found at www.cdisc.org.

HIPAA

HIPAA is the Health Insurance Portability and Accountability Act of 1996. It is a federal law. Like 21 CFR it covers quite a range of topics. The sections that most apply to data management are those on privacy (see 45 CFR Parts 160 and 164 for the actual rule).

The rules apply to covered entities that are generally people such as your private physician or organizations like medical centers or research hospitals. Those entities may not transfer identifiable data to another organization without explicit permission from the patient for each transfer. So why are sponsors of clinical trials able to receive datasets that identify each patient, albeit without a name? The rule has provisions for research. Those provisions require the consent of the patient for the purpose of a single study. The informed-consent document that patients sign in clinical trials serves this purpose.

Data management groups that work with research institutions occasionally get calls from those sites asking that some data fields be removed from the case report form. Most often the field in question is the birth date. Some sites request that only the year be provided. The database design must handle partial birth dates should the sponsor not be able to convince the institution that the data is permitted. Patient initials are another kind of identifying field that may be called into question.

Data managers can attend short introductions to HIPAA offered by a wide range of groups and private instructors. The National Institutes of Health publishes useful material to explain the rule and its impact on clinical research. In particular, refer to its Web publication, "Clinical Research and the HIPAA Privacy Rule," and other useful materials found at: http://privacyruleandresearch.nih.gov/clin_research.asp.

Index

A